THE EVERYTHING®
METABOLISM
DIET COOKBOOK

Dear Reader,

Have you ever found yourself blaming your metabolism ("I just can't lose weight no matter what I do. My metabolism is too slow") or crediting someone else's metabolism ("She's lucky she has a fast metabolism. She can eat whatever she wants and not gain weight") for the difference in ability or inability to lose weight? If so, you're not alone. In fact, I was right there with you for a long time.

I had lumped myself into the category of people with a slow metabolism. I figured if I wanted to lose weight and keep it off, I would have to work much harder than most. Eventually, however, I realized that this wasn't the case. I didn't have to work harder. I just had to work smarter.

Your metabolism is not fixed; it's dynamic, which means it's constantly changing. This is an enormous benefit when it comes to weight loss—and health in general—because it means that the daily choices you make have a tremendous impact on how your metabolism is functioning.

Your body composition (how much fat versus muscle you have), your hormones, and your stress and activity levels all largely affect your metabolism—which puts the power in your hands. You have the ability to change your body composition, balance your hormones, reduce your stress, and increase your activity levels, all by making different daily choices.

Turning your metabolism into an efficient calorie-burning machine is not something that happens overnight, but the journey is well worth it. I hope you'll join me.

I wish you all the best in health and in life.

Lindsay Boyers, CHNC

Welcome to the EVERYTHING® Series!

These handy, accessible books give you all you need to tackle a difficult project, gain a new hobby, comprehend a fascinating topic, prepare for an exam, or even brush up on something you learned back in school but have since forgotten.

You can choose to read an Everything® book from cover to cover or just pick out the information you want from our four useful boxes: e-questions, e-facts, e-alerts, and e-ssentials.

We give you everything you need to know on the subject, but throw in a lot of fun stuff along the way, too.

We now have more than 400 Everything® books in print, spanning such wide-ranging categories as weddings, pregnancy, cooking, music instruction, foreign language, crafts, pets, New Age, and so much more. When you're done reading them all, you can finally say you know Everything®!

QUESTION

Answers to common questions

FACT

Important snippets of information

ALERT

Urgent warnings

ESSENTIAL

Quick handy tips

PUBLISHER Karen Cooper

MANAGING EDITOR, EVERYTHING® SERIES Lisa Laing

COPY CHIEF Casey Ebert

ASSISTANT PRODUCTION EDITOR Alex Guarco

ACQUISITIONS EDITOR Hillary Thompson

SENIOR DEVELOPMENT EDITOR Brett Palana-Shanahan

EVERYTHING® SERIES COVER DESIGNER Erin Alexander

Visit the entire Everything® series at *www.everything.com*

THE EVERYTHING METABOLISM DIET COOKBOOK

Lindsay Boyers, CHNC

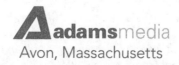

Adamsmedia

Avon, Massachusetts

To Tiffany
I could never put into words how much you mean to me and
how lucky I am to have you as a big sister. I love you, B.

An Everything® Series Book.
Everything® and everything.com® are registered trademarks of F+W Media, Inc.

Published by
Adams Media, a division of F+W Media, Inc.
57 Littlefield Street, Avon, MA 02322. U.S.A.
www.adamsmedia.com

ISBN 10: 1-4405-9228-4
ISBN 13: 978-1-4405-9228-7
eISBN 10: 1-4405-9229-2
eISBN 13: 978-1-4405-9229-4

Printed in the United States of America.

10 9 8 7 6 5 4 3 2 1

The information in this book should not be used for diagnosing or treating any health problem. Not all diet and exercise plans suit everyone. You should always consult a trained medical professional before starting a diet, taking any form of medication, or embarking on any fitness or weight-training program. The author and publisher disclaim any liability arising directly or indirectly from the use of this book.

Always follow safety and commonsense cooking protocol while using kitchen utensils, operating ovens and stoves, and handling uncooked food. If children are assisting in the preparation of any recipe, they should always be supervised by an adult.

Many of the designations used by manufacturers and sellers to distinguish their products are claimed as trademarks. Where those designations appear in this book and F+W Media, Inc. was aware of a trademark claim, the designations have been printed with initial capital letters.

Cover images © StockFood/Keller & Keller Photography; StockFood/Comet, Renée; StockFood/Meridith, Marla; StockFood/Ranek, Lars.

This book is available at quantity discounts for bulk purchases.
For information, please call 1-800-289-0963.

Contents

Acknowledgments

Thank you to my family—my mom, Lola; my dad, Scott; my sister, Tiffany; and my brother, Sean—for always being in my corner and supporting me no matter what I'm doing. I couldn't have handpicked a better family and I love you all.

Thank you also to Hillary Thompson for giving me this opportunity and answering my questions along the way.

Introduction

IN TODAY'S WORLD, IT'S commonplace to abuse your body. The combination of processed foods, high-stress lifestyles, and little time to unwind that has become the norm is a recipe for disaster. Eventually, this toxic combo takes a toll on your body—and then enters misplaced blame.

When you find that you've gained weight, but have trouble losing it, you immediately point the finger at your metabolism with seemingly innocent phrases like "I just can't lose weight no matter what I do. I have a slow metabolism." That might be true at this moment, but was it always that way? And does it have to stay that way? The answer to both of these questions is no.

Many people think metabolism is a fixed thing and there's really nothing you can do to change it, but this isn't true. Your metabolism isn't static. It's constantly changing and evolving based on the feedback it receives from your body. What you're eating, how much you're moving, how you're handling your stress levels, and your general attitude all affect the state of your metabolism.

Years of bad choices—processed and nutrient-poor foods, not enough sleep, too little exercise, exposure to toxins in your food and your self-care products, and a fast-paced lifestyle have all contributed to the state your metabolism is in right now. These choices have literally changed your biochemistry by changing the hormonal signaling in your body.

This was a gradual change—something that happened over time. You may not have noticed it until you stopped for a minute and actually took a look at yourself in the mirror. All of a sudden you're overweight, tired, and moody. You can barely make it through lunch without wanting to put your head down for a nap at your desk at work. You can't go on like this. Something has to change.

The problem is you may not know where to start. Luckily, just like years of bad choices have altered your metabolism to the state it's in now, making good choices can get it back to where it needs to be for you to reach your ideal weight and experience energy and clarity like never before.

Providing your body with whole and nutrient-dense foods, exercising regularly, getting enough sleep, and taking steps to reduce your stress doesn't just feel good; it alters your hormones and brings your body back to a state of homeostasis—or balance. Your body wants to function optimally and healthily, it just has a hard time doing so when it doesn't have the right tools.

This transformation doesn't happen overnight; just like it took time to get to where you are now, it can take some time to get your metabolism back to where it's supposed to be. The good news is that within only a few days of treating your body right, you'll begin to experience changes that will motivate you to stay on track. Maybe you're less bloated and your pants fit a little better, or you're able to get out of bed in the morning without hitting that snooze button several times, or your skin appears brighter and softer—these are all indications that your hormones are getting back on track and you're on your way to having a healthy, happy metabolism. When you start being good to your body, it will thank you by being good to you.

CHAPTER 1

Understanding Metabolism

The term "metabolism" gets thrown around a lot. You've probably heard something like, "I can't lose weight because I have a slow metabolism," or, "You're so lucky that you have such a fast metabolism. You can eat whatever you want without gaining weight!" While these statements do indicate a basic understanding of part of what your metabolism does—controls your weight—it's really just the beginning. Your metabolism is so much more than that. It's not a single "thing" as some people describe it; rather, it's all the chemical processes that occur within you that keep you alive.

What Is Metabolism?

To put it simply, metabolism is a blanket term that describes all the chemical reactions that help convert the food you eat into energy that your body can use for a wide range of activities, like moving, thinking, growing, and sleeping. Every second, there are thousands of metabolic reactions occurring in your body at the same time. All of these metabolic activities can be categorized into two major types: catabolic and anabolic.

Types of Metabolism

Catabolic metabolism refers to the breakdown of food components into simpler forms to produce energy. The food you eat is not in a form that your body can use. This is where catabolic metabolism comes into play—it takes proteins, fats, and carbohydrates and breaks them down into amino acids, fatty acids, and glucose—the components that your body can use for energy.

Once catabolic metabolism has done its job, anabolic metabolism takes over. Anabolic metabolism takes the components left from catabolic metabolism and uses them to build cells and body tissues. Some components may also be stored as energy for later use.

FACT

Catabolic reactions release energy that is used to drive all chemical reactions. This energy is stored as ATP—or adenosine triphosphate. The human body only contains about 9 ounces (250 grams) of ATP at a time, but this ATP is continuously recycled and reused.

Both types of metabolism are controlled by hormones. Like metabolism, the hormones that play a role in weight and metabolism are either categorized as catabolic or anabolic hormones. You need both catabolic and anabolic hormones for your metabolism to function properly. The key is to maintain the proper balance of these hormones through a proper diet and lifestyle practices.

The Major Hormones

Your hormones are chemical messengers that control all of the reactions in your body. The purpose of your hormonal, or endocrine, system is to maintain homeostasis—or a perfect equilibrium—of your body. When blood levels of certain hormones go down, endocrine glands respond by making and releasing more of that hormone. When blood levels of hormones go up, endocrine glands respond by decreasing hormonal production. In a healthy body, this system works without a hitch. In a body that's undernourished, overstressed, and overtaxed by environmental toxicity, this delicate hormonal balance can get thrown way off.

Insulin

Insulin is one of the most commonly discussed hormones and one of the major players in your metabolism. Insulin's primary function is to lower your blood sugar by attaching to the glucose molecules in your blood and carrying them to your cells. Shortly after you eat a meal, especially a meal that's high in refined carbohydrates, glucose is released into your bloodstream and your blood sugar rises. In response to this rise in blood sugar, your pancreas—an organ located just behind your stomach—releases insulin into your bloodstream.

Insulin does one of three things—it carries glucose to the cells to use immediately for energy, it carries glucose to the liver where it's converted to glycogen and stored for use as energy at a time when your body doesn't have access to glucose from a meal, or it helps convert glucose into fatty acids that are then stored as fat in your fat cells. Your body calls on the energy from these fatty acids in the absence of glucose, which is part of the point of this program.

How Insulin Gets Out of Whack

Problems with insulin occur when your body stops effectively responding to it. Why does this happen? The simple answer is overexposure. When you eat a lot of refined carbohydrates—pasta, bread, desserts, sugar—your blood sugar is chronically high. As a result, your pancreas pumps out excess amounts of insulin to try to compensate for this high blood sugar level. Insulin sweeps up the glucose in record time and carries it out of your blood, which causes your blood sugar to drop and leaves you feeling hungry and craving more refined carbohydrates.

ESSENTIAL

The Centers for Disease Control and Prevention estimates that 29.1 million people in the United States are currently living with diabetes and that almost 30 percent of people with diabetes don't even know they have it. If you suspect insulin resistance, it's important to get your hormone levels under control so that it does not progress into diabetes.

While your body may be able to handle this cycle at first, eventually the cells stop responding effectively to the excess insulin. Now, it's not just your blood sugar that's high; it's your insulin levels as well. This is called insulin resistance—and it's a major precursor to type 2 diabetes and metabolic syndrome.

Signs of Insulin Imbalance

Your body is pretty good at letting you know when something isn't right, and hormonal imbalance is no exception. Some common signs of insulin imbalance include:

- Abdominal obesity
- Acne
- Blurred vision
- Dark patches of skin on body creases (armpits, groin, neck)
- Depression
- Difficulty falling or staying asleep
- Fatigue
- Inability to lose weight
- Increased thirst
- Increased urination

Thyroid

Next up are your thyroid hormones, which are major metabolic players. Your thyroid gland is a butterfly-shaped organ that's located just below the Adam's apple (or where the Adam's apple would be) and above the collarbone. Your thyroid takes the mineral iodine and converts it into two different thyroid hormones: T3 (triiodothyronine) and T4 (thyroxine). These hormones are then released into the blood where they control metabolism—or the conversion of calories to energy. Every single cell in your body relies on these thyroid hormones for metabolism. A healthy, functioning thyroid gland produces about 80 percent T4 and 20 percent T3. T3 possesses four times the hormonal strength of T4.

The thyroid gland is controlled by the pituitary gland—a pea-sized gland that sits at the base of the brain. The pituitary gland produces thyroid-stimulating hormone (TSH), which signals the thyroid to release its hormones in response to lowered levels in the blood.

How Thyroid Hormones Get Out of Whack

Your thyroid is sensitive to chronic stress, nutritional deprivation, environmental toxins, extreme dieting, certain medications, and inflammatory disease processes. If any or all of these are present, your thyroid may respond by shutting down or speeding up. As a result, you can end up hypothyroid (too few thyroid hormones) or hyperthyroid (too many thyroid hormones).

ALERT

Thyroid imbalance can be a serious problem. If you suspect either an overactive or underactive thyroid, make an appointment with your healthcare provider to get your thyroid levels checked.

Signs of Thyroid Imbalance

Some common signs that you have too little thyroid hormones include:

- Brain fog
- Coarse hair and skin
- Confusion

- Constipation
- Depression
- Difficulty swallowing
- Dry skin
- Fatigue
- Heavy periods
- Intolerance to cold
- Loss of hair
- Muscle cramps
- Slow pulse
- Weight gain

Some common signs that you have too much thyroid hormone include:

- Diarrhea
- Dizziness
- Fatigue
- Hyperactivity
- Increased pulse
- Increased sweating
- Insomnia
- Irritability
- Nervousness/anxiety
- Weight loss

Fight-or-Flight Hormones

Your fight-or-flight response is designed to save your life in times of immediate danger. Think about it this way: In ancient times, your ancestors had to hunt and gather for food. Occasionally, they would run into something life-threatening, like a tiger. In that split second of having to make a decision of whether to fight the tiger or to run away from it, the body releases the hormones norepinephrine, epinephrine, and cortisol.

Norepinephrine signals the body to stop producing insulin. The purpose of this is to allow glucose to remain in the blood so that you have access to a quick source of energy should you need it. Epinephrine stops digestion and relaxes the muscles of the stomach and intestines to decrease blood flow to these areas. The purpose of this is to allow more blood to flow to the extremities so that you can more effectively fight or run. Once the immediate stress is over, cortisol signals your body to stop pumping out norepinephrine and epinephrine and to resume normal function.

FACT

In humans, the normal secretion of cortisol follows a diurnal (or daily) cycle. Cortisol levels are naturally increased right after awakening and then decrease as the day goes on. In someone with cortisol imbalance, this natural cycle may be flipped, causing increased cortisol levels at night and decreased levels first thing in the morning.

While this hormonal response is extremely useful in stressful situations when you need to act fast, it's become a problem due to the chronic stress of today's lifestyle. Many people live in a chronic fight-or-flight state, which translates to high cortisol levels. This is a problem because cortisol is a catabolic hormone, which means that it breaks things down. Excess cortisol breaks down muscle, bone, and skin and can lead to osteoporosis and stretch marks. Cortisol also signals your body to store fat in your abdomen. This is why high stress levels are associated with excess belly fat.

How Stress Hormones Get Out of Whack

Chronic stress—from a poor diet, being overworked, and not relaxing enough—overstimulates the adrenals, which are the glands that lie on top of your kidneys and produce these hormones. Long-term activation of this stress response leads to a sensitization to stress. Over time, this feedback loop becomes stronger and stronger and even minor threats will cause a major stress response.

Signs of Cortisol Imbalance

Some common signs of cortisol imbalance include:

- Anxiety
- Belly fat
- Depression

- Diarrhea
- Easily bruised skin
- Fatigue
- High/low blood pressure
- Insomnia
- Insulin resistance
- Irregular periods
- Loss of appetite
- Salt cravings
- Weight gain/weight loss

The Steroid Hormones

The steroid hormones, sometimes referred to as the sex hormones, include estrogen, progesterone, testosterone, and dehydroepiandrosterone (DHEA). Although estrogen and progesterone are most often associated with women and testosterone and DHEA are most often associated with men, both men and women have both—just in different balances. The key to keeping the metabolism running smoothly is to maintain that ideal balance in your own body.

Estrogen and Progesterone

Estrogen has a wide range of roles—especially in a woman's body. Estrogen impacts development, digestion, heart function, electrolyte balance, memory, and bone density. There are many different types of estrogen in a woman's body, but the three main types are estradiol, estrone, and estriol. Estradiol is more prominent in younger women. It helps lower insulin and blood pressure and helps keep a woman's body lean. It also regulates hunger, mood, and energy levels. As you age, the production of estradiol decreases and estrone becomes the main estrogen hormone. Estrone signals your body to hold onto fat. Estriol is a waste product of the metabolism of estradiol. Compared to estradiol and estrone, estriol has weak estrogenic activity.

In men, when estrogen is in balance with testosterone, it has little effect on metabolism. But if estrogen levels become too high, it can decrease lean muscle mass and lead to fat storage.

How Estrogen Gets Out of Whack

Many people write off problems with estrogen as an unavoidable part of getting older. While it's true that the levels of hormones shift as you age, you can change your fate with the choices you make. There are many chemicals that mimic the activity of estrogen. When you're exposed to these chemicals, your body thinks that estrogen levels are rising and it responds accordingly—by increasing fat storage, decreasing libido, and causing depression/anxiety, to name a few. So where are these chemicals coming from? They're the preservatives in your food, the fragrance in your perfume, and the synthetic chemicals in your kitchen cleaner. They're literally all around you.

Signs of Estrogen Imbalance

Some common signs of estrogen imbalance in women include:

- Anxiety
- Belly fat/bloating
- Brain fog
- Carbohydrate cravings
- Decreased libido
- Depression
- Dizziness
- Dry skin
- Fatigue
- Hair loss
- PMS/PMDD

Some signs of estrogen imbalance in men include:

- Decreased libido
- Decreased muscle tone
- Depression
- Erectile dysfunction
- Excess breast tissue
- Increased body fat
- Low sperm count

Testosterone and DHEA

Testosterone and DHEA are androgen hormones, which are anabolic hormones by definition. They build instead of destroy—and usually it's muscle. Testosterone helps increase lean muscle mass, build strength, improve libido, and increase energy in both sexes. Most of the testosterone and DHEA in a man's body comes from the testes. In a women's body, testosterone and DHEA come from the adrenal glands.

How Androgens Get Out of Whack

As you age, your body naturally starts to decrease its production of both testosterone and DHEA. What happens next is a Catch-22. The decrease of the androgen hormones leads to increased fat storage and decreased motivation to exercise. Increased fat storage causes your body to convert testosterone to estrogen, further reducing levels. Combine advancing age with a nutrient-poor, refined carbohydrate–rich diet, and your testosterone and DHEA have no chance.

Signs of Androgen Hormone Imbalance

Some common signs of androgen hormone imbalance in include:

- Acne
- Aggression
- Anxiety
- Belly fat
- Changes in body composition
- Decreased libido
- Depression
- Erectile dysfunction
- Fatigue
- Hair loss
- Lowered voice
- Reduced bone density

Ghrelin and Leptin

Ghrelin and leptin are the hunger hormones. Ghrelin is released by the stomach and small intestine. It tells your body when you're hungry. In someone with a healthy, functioning metabolism, ghrelin increases when you haven't eaten in a while and decreases as you start to fill up.

Leptin does the opposite of ghrelin. Leptin lets you know when it's time to stop eating. It signals the brain that the body has enough fat stores. The problem is that when you're overweight or your metabolism is out of whack, your body doesn't respond to leptin effectively, even if you have higher levels of leptin in the blood. As a result, you never feel full no matter how much you've eaten.

How Leptin and Ghrelin Get Out of Whack

So what causes these hormones to become imbalanced? You guessed it: your lifestyle. The major issue here is an imbalance with leptin, but surprisingly, low levels of leptin aren't usually the problem. In fact, researchers have discovered that people with a higher body fat percentage tend to have higher levels of leptin in the blood. The problem is that when you're constantly overeating—or eating foods that are high in the wrong carbohydrates or trans fats—not getting enough sleep, and living a life full of chronic stress, the receptors in your brain that are supposed to respond to leptin don't. This is called leptin resistance—and it goes hand in hand with insulin resistance.

Signs of Leptin Resistance

Some common signs of leptin resistance include:

- Constant hunger
- Depression
- Diabetes
- High blood pressure
- Inflammation
- Obesity

How Did You Get Here?

If any of the symptoms and hormonal issues sound like you, you're probably left wondering how you got to this place and, more importantly, what you can do about it. First, you need to understand the "how" so that you can effectively implement the lifestyle changes that will get your metabolism back on track. Many people want to immediately blame genetics, but that's only a piece of the puzzle—and sometimes a minor one. Genetics do play a role in what's going on in your body, but researchers estimate that that role is only 10–30 percent, depending on the condition. Have you ever heard the phrase "Your genes load the gun, and your environment/choices pull the trigger"? The take-home message is that even if you're predisposed to something because of your genetic makeup, the way that you live your life has a dramatic impact on which genes express and which ones don't.

Poor Diet

Some of the foods available today are an absolute nightmare when it comes to a properly functioning metabolism. Why is that? Because your body doesn't even recognize commercially produced, processed foods as food. These foods are made in a lab—they contain artificial ingredients, preservatives, excess amounts of sugar, and genetically modified organisms (GMO). The more processed a food is, the more damage it can do to your biochemistry. On another note, these processed foods are not only unrecognizable as food, they're also low in the nutrients your body needs to thrive. Some manufacturers try to get around this by fortifying processed foods with vitamins and minerals, but your body is only able to absorb a fraction of these synthetic compounds.

FACT

One animal study found that natural vitamin B_1 was absorbed 1.38 times more effectively than an isolated synthetic vitamin B_1 compound. Vitamin B_2 was absorbed 1.92 times more effectively, and vitamin B_3 was absorbed 3.94 times more effectively.

Along with poor diet comes a history of extreme, or yo-yo, dieting. Extreme dieting—like very-low-calorie diets, prolonged juicing, or cleanse-type diets that don't offer the proper nutritional support—disrupts your hormonal balance by sending messages to your metabolism to slow down in case this "famine" persists and food is no longer plentiful. Starvation diets are catabolic, which means they trigger your body to break down your muscles for energy. When you lose lean muscle mass, your body becomes less effective at burning calories at rest, so you end up having to work harder to lose weight.

Not Enough Exercise

It's true that the production of some of your hormones declines as you age, but more research is pointing to the fact that you actually have more control over this decline than you think. In addition to the proper diet, exercise helps balance hormones naturally and helps increase lean muscle mass. Every pound of muscle that you have burns three times more calories than every pound of fat. That means as you build more lean muscle and lose body fat, your metabolism becomes more efficient.

QUESTION

What types of exercise should I do?
Incorporate all forms of exercise into your weekly routine. Combining cardiovascular exercise, like jogging, with strength-training exercise, like lifting weights, and stress-reducing exercise, like yoga or tai chi, provides the most benefit for hormone balance.

On the other hand, lack of exercise translates to increased body fat, lowered hormone levels, and metabolism disruption.

Too Much Stress—and Not Enough Stress Relief

Even just a little bit of prolonged stress can significantly disrupt your hormones. This stress-related hormonal disruption is associated with a decreased metabolism and weight gain. It's true that you cannot completely avoid stress, but it's important to take steps to manage your stress levels every day.

Too Little Sleep

Alongside too much stress comes not enough sleep. As your stress levels rise, you begin to sacrifice sleep to get your work done. Maybe you're getting up too early to fit some exercise in or maybe you're going to bed too late to meet that important deadline. Maybe the overthinking associated with stress has led to insomnia or an inability to get a restful night's sleep. Whatever the reason, a lack of adequate sleep is one of the biggest causes of hormonal disruption related to stress.

When you're sleep deprived, your body produces more ghrelin and less leptin. As a result, your body is constantly telling you to eat without letting you know that it's time to stop. Your metabolism also slows down when you haven't had a good night of sleep so you're not using the calories you are eating as efficiently.

Environmental Toxicity

Environmental toxicity is a major player in hormonal and metabolism disruption that doesn't get talked about nearly enough. There are almost 100,000 synthetic chemicals that are registered for commercial use, with thousands more being added each year. These synthetic chemicals are found in processed foods, cosmetics, skincare products, household cleaning items, plastics, etc. The problem is that most of these synthetic chemicals have never even been tested for safety—and a large amount of those that have, have been found to be endocrine disrupting. That means that even at very low levels, exposure to these synthetic chemicals can throw off your hormonal balance. This can cause health issues across the board, including weight gain, autoimmune diseases like asthma and Hashimoto's thyroiditis, allergic reactions, and cancer.

Metabolism Diet Breakdown

Now that you know the how, it's time to delve into what you can do about it. The good news is that the answer is simple: treat your body right. That being said, just because something is *simple* doesn't necessarily make it *easy*. It's likely that you're going to have to unlearn years of bad habits, but just take it day by day and breathe. The more you follow these healthy habits, the more they will become part of your lifestyle.

The Diet Stages

This program is divided into three separate stages, but unlike other diet programs that require you to remain in each step for a specified number of weeks or months, you'll cycle through each stage every week. Stage 1 lasts for three days, then you move on to Stage 2 for two days, and Stage 3 for two days. Every week, you'll progress through all three stages and then begin Stage 1 again.

Stage 1

Stage 1 is all about calming down your adrenal glands and getting your stress hormones under control. It's rich in carbohydrates from healthy grains, like quinoa, wild rice, and oatmeal, and natural sugars from fruit. You'll also be getting a hefty dose of B vitamins, which help reduce stress levels. Stage 1 also allows moderate amounts of protein, but only low amounts of fat.

The goal of this stage is to give the body the nutrients it needs, without putting stress on the adrenals by causing major spikes and drops in blood sugar levels.

Stage 1 is also designed to stimulate digestive enzymes that allow you to properly break down the food you are eating so that your body has access to the vitamins, minerals, and phytonutrients and can use them to repair your body and your metabolism. Everything you eat on Stage 1—and all the stages for that matter—will be nutrient-dense and unprocessed.

Stage 2

Stage 2 is about stimulating your body to release the fat from your fat stores to use as energy. Stage 2 is high in lean proteins and foods that support liver function, so it can help your body burn more stored fat. In order to turn your body from using glucose as energy to burning fat for fuel, this stage allows no fruit or grains. The purpose of this is to eliminate foods that significantly elevate your blood sugar and tax your hormonal system.

Stage 3

In Stage 3, you get the best of both worlds—healthy grains and healthy fats in addition to protein. Although the grains and fruits you can enjoy on Stage 3 are slightly more limited than on Stage 1, there are still plenty of choices. The goal of Stage 3 is to stoke your metabolism and really get it to burn calories effectively. The foods you eat during Stage 3 target your hormones and heart while increasing your metabolic heat. Stage 3 is the high-fat, moderate-protein, and low-glycemic stage.

In addition to the comprehensive recipes in this book, you'll also find detailed food lists that outline exactly what's allowed in each stage and what's not. There's also a master list of foods that are excluded from all stages. In general, you should try to choose organic foods whenever possible. Conventional and GMO foods contain pesticides that fall under the category of environmental toxicity. When you're working to balance these hormones, exposing yourself to endocrine-disrupting pesticides can negate all of your hard work.

Other Rules

It's not just what you eat, but also when you eat and how you eat, that affects how your body responds to food. Because of that, there are a few other guidelines to follow when participating in this program.

You must eat three meals per day and at least one snack. As your metabolism starts to adjust, you may start to feel less hungry, but you still need to get all your meals in. Breakfast must be eaten within one hour of waking up. Drink a glass of water—ideally room temperature water with a squeeze of fresh lemon—immediately upon waking. Eat slowly and mindfully. Avoid all distractions and give your meal the proper attention it deserves. Chew each bite carefully and savor the meal. After all, it's doing the important job of nourishing your body.

Other Major Players

What you're eating is extremely important to your health, but it's not the only piece of the puzzle. While following this diet plan, there are other things you can (and should) do to maximize your success and help rebalance your hormones.

Move Your Body

Exercise dramatically affects your body composition and your hormones by reducing cortisol and making your cells more sensitive to insulin. Exercise also increases DHEA and boosts endorphins—the feel-good biochemicals that enhance your mood and help you control stress. Make it a goal to exercise for thirty minutes to an hour every day. Choose exercises that will get your heart pumping, and include strength training to help increase your lean muscle mass.

Get Enough Sleep

Nowadays, people tend to glorify being busy—and this comes at the expense of health. Sleep should be a priority, not a luxury. Make it a goal to get between seven and nine hours every night. Anything under seven hours can disrupt those hunger hormones and contribute to metabolic disruption.

Relieve Your Stress

Stress is inevitable. You may not be able to completely avoid it, but you can manage it—and it's vital that you do. Get a weekly massage and do yoga twice a week. Learn to meditate and write your experiences down in a journal. Connect with friends more often and remove toxic people from your life. Reduce your workload by asking for help or delegating tasks. Do something that you enjoy—write, draw, read, or ride a bike. Make it a point to go outside and enjoy nature for an hour a day. Practice deep breathing. There are a multitude of things that you can do to reduce your stress levels. Experiment until you find what works for you.

CHAPTER 2

MD Stage 1 Breakfast

Apple-Cinnamon Quinoa Porridge

Quinoa is often thought of as a savory dinnertime side, but it can also make a warm, comforting breakfast dish that you can eat in place of traditional oatmeal.

INGREDIENTS | SERVES 2

½ cup quinoa
1 small Granny Smith apple, cored and diced
¾ cup water
1 teaspoon ground cinnamon
⅛ teaspoon salt

Make It Yours!

This recipe is a basic template for quinoa porridge. You can make it your own by replacing the apple and cinnamon with any other Stage 1–approved items. Try blueberries and ginger or strawberries and nutmeg.

1. Rinse quinoa with cold water until water runs clear. Drain quinoa in a fine strainer or cheesecloth.

2. Combine all ingredients in a medium saucepan over medium-high heat. Bring mixture to a boil and then reduce heat to low.

3. Cook covered 15–20 minutes or until water is absorbed and quinoa is soft.

4. Remove from heat and let sit covered 5 minutes. Fluff with a fork and divide mixture evenly between two bowls. Serve warm.

Peach Pear Smoothie

You can kick this smoothie up a notch by also adding some freshly grated ginger, but remember—a little goes a long way!

INGREDIENTS | SERVES 2

⅓ cup frozen peaches
⅓ cup frozen pears
¼ teaspoon ground cinnamon
1 cup coconut water
1 tablespoon fresh lemon juice
1 cup fresh spinach

Put all ingredients in a blender and blend until smooth.

Overnight Oats

This recipe must be prepared in advance, so make sure to plan accordingly when you want to eat it for breakfast.

INGREDIENTS | SERVES 2

½ cup steel-cut oats

½ cup strawberries

½ cup blueberries

¼ teaspoon ground cinnamon

⅛ teaspoon ground nutmeg

2 cups water

Steel-Cut versus Old-Fashioned: What's the Big Deal?

This recipe calls specifically for steel-cut oats—and there's a reason for that. Steel-cut oats are the least processed type of oat cereal, and because of this they have a lower glycemic index than other types of oats. This means they won't raise your blood sugar as significantly.

1. Place oats, berries, cinnamon, and nutmeg in a large bowl and toss together. Cover mixture with water and stir until combined.

2. Cover and let mixture sit in the refrigerator overnight. In the morning, remove mixture from refrigerator and heat in a medium saucepan over low heat 20 minutes, stirring occasionally.

3. Serve warm.

Spirulina Power Smoothie

This Spirulina Power Smoothie is sure to start your day off right. It's loaded with protein and micronutrients and will keep you full until lunch.

INGREDIENTS | SERVES 2

1 cup water
1 small cucumber, sliced
1 small green apple, cored and sliced
½ cup frozen mixed berries
2 teaspoons spirulina
1 teaspoon granulated stevia (optional)

Combine all ingredients in a blender and blend until smooth.

Spirulina: The Green Superfood

Spirulina has earned its rightful place as a superfood. The natural algae is 65 percent protein and a good source of antioxidants, B vitamins, and several other vitamins and minerals. The chlorophyll in spirulina, which gives it its green color, helps cleanse the blood and boost the immune system.

Mango Pineapple Smoothie

This recipe calls for fresh fruit, but you may substitute frozen if you wish. If you do, you may need to add extra water until you reach your desired consistency.

INGREDIENTS | SERVES 2

½ cup cubed fresh mango
½ cup cubed fresh pineapple
3 tablespoons fresh lemon juice
1 cup ice cubes
1 cup water

Combine all ingredients in a blender and blend until smooth.

Blueberry French Toast

You can adjust this French toast to your liking by replacing the blueberries with any Stage 1–approved fruit. You can try mixed berries, strawberries, peaches, pears, or apples, for example.

INGREDIENTS | SERVES 2

1 cup frozen blueberries
1 tablespoon lemon juice
¼ teaspoon stevia powder
⅛ teaspoon salt
2 large egg whites
2 teaspoons vanilla extract
½ teaspoon ground cinnamon
2 slices sprouted-grain bread

Sprouted Grain versus Unsprouted Grain

For this recipe, make sure to use sprouted wheat or grain bread, which is usually found in the freezer section of the grocery store. Sprouted grains contain less gluten and more protein than regular grains. They are also easier to digest.

1. Put blueberries in a small saucepan and heat over medium heat until blueberries start to bubble and burst, about 5 minutes. Add lemon juice, stevia, and salt and stir until fruit mixture reaches desired consistency. Set aside.

2. Whisk egg whites, vanilla, and cinnamon together in a small bowl. Soak each sprouted-bread slice in the mixture, making sure to coat both sides.

3. Transfer bread to a medium skillet and cook over medium heat, flipping once so that both sides are browned.

4. Transfer French toast to a plate and top each slice with half the blueberry mixture. Serve warm.

Chicken Apple Sausage with Scrambled Egg Whites

*For this recipe, you can use any chicken sausage that doesn't contain added sugar
or corn syrup, or replace the sausage with sugar-free turkey bacon.*

INGREDIENTS | SERVES 2

1 teaspoon water

1 (3-ounce) chicken apple sausage
link (no sugar added), chopped into
small pieces

1 cup chopped spinach

4 large egg whites

¼ teaspoon garlic salt

¼ teaspoon ground black pepper

1. Heat water over medium heat in a small skillet. Add sausage and toss in heated skillet, stirring occasionally until sausage is browned. Once sausage is browned, add spinach to the pan and cook until wilted, about 3 minutes.

2. In a separate medium bowl, whisk together egg whites, garlic salt, and pepper. Pour egg mixture over sausage mixture and scramble until cooked, about 3–4 minutes.

3. Serve warm.

Blueberry-Lemon Quinoa Porridge

Don't skip the lemon zest in this recipe! The zest gives this breakfast porridge a powerful flavor boost. For some extra kick, you can add a little freshly grated ginger.

INGREDIENTS | SERVES 2

½ cup quinoa

1 cup water

⅛ teaspoon salt

Zest from ½ large lemon

½ cup blueberries

1 teaspoon ground flaxseed

1 teaspoon granulated stevia

Don't Skip the Rinse!

Many packaged quinoas are prerinsed, but follow this step anyway. Rinsing the quinoa removes the outer coating, called saponin, which can give the quinoa a bitter or soapy taste.

1. Rinse quinoa under cold water until water runs clear. Strain quinoa with a fine-mesh strainer or cheesecloth.

2. Combine quinoa and water in a medium saucepan and bring to a boil over high heat. Once mixture starts boiling, add salt, reduce heat to low, cover, and allow to simmer until all water is absorbed, about 20 minutes.

3. Remove saucepan from heat and fluff quinoa with a fork. Add lemon zest, blueberries, flaxseed, and stevia. Serve warm.

Metabolism-Boosting Smoothie

This recipe calls for unsweetened green tea, not the sugar-laden bottled varieties. It's best to steep an organic green tea bag in ½ cup of water for 4 minutes just before preparing the smoothie.

INGREDIENTS | SERVES 2

1 cup coconut water

½ cup unsweetened green iced tea

¼ cup broccoli florets

1 cup frozen strawberries

¼ cup canned cannellini beans, drained and rinsed

½ teaspoon granulated stevia

½ teaspoon ground cinnamon

⅛ teaspoon ground ginger

Combine all ingredients in a blender and blend until smooth.

The Power of Green Tea

Green tea not only promotes fat oxidation—or the breakdown of fat—it also has thermogenic properties, which means it may speed up metabolism. Thermogenesis refers to the amount of calories the body burns during digestion and absorption.

Breakfast Stuffed Sweet Potatoes

Sweet potatoes and eggs are such a wonderful combination. You can bring out the sweetness of the sweet potato by sprinkling it with a little bit of cinnamon prior to piling the eggs on top.

INGREDIENTS | SERVES 2

1 medium sweet potato, cut in half lengthwise
2 teaspoons water
½ teaspoon minced garlic
¼ cup chopped yellow onion
1 cup chopped spinach
4 large egg whites
½ teaspoon salt
¼ teaspoon ground black pepper
½ teaspoon onion powder

1. Preheat oven to 400°F. Place sweet potato cut-side down on a baking sheet. Bake in oven 25 minutes or until sweet potato is soft.

2. When sweet potato is done cooking, heat water in a medium skillet over medium heat. Add garlic and onion and cook until soft, about 5 minutes. Add spinach and cook until wilted, about 3 minutes.

3. In a medium bowl, whisk egg whites with salt, pepper, and onion powder. Pour egg mixture over spinach mixture and scramble until eggs are cooked through. Remove from heat.

4. Mash the sweet potato flesh with a fork inside the potato skin. Top each sweet potato half with half the egg mixture. Serve warm.

Amaranth Breakfast Porridge

It's important not to overcook this Amaranth Breakfast Porridge. If you cook the grain too long, it can turn to mush. You'll know it's done when it's soft but you can still see the individual grain pieces.

INGREDIENTS | SERVES 2

1 cup water
½ cup amaranth
½ teaspoon ground cinnamon
¼ teaspoon ground allspice
1 teaspoon granulated stevia
½ cup fresh blueberries

1. Mix water and amaranth in a small saucepan and bring to a boil over high heat. Reduce heat to low and simmer 20 minutes or until most of the water is absorbed. Do not overcook.

2. Mix in cinnamon, allspice, and stevia. Transfer to two serving bowls and top with fresh blueberries. Serve immediately.

Amaranth Gets an A+

Amaranth contains more than three times the average amount of calcium of other grains. It's also high in magnesium, phosphorus, and potassium, and it's the only grain source of vitamin C. Amaranth also contains 13–14 percent protein, significantly more than other grains.

Oatmeal Smoothie

This smoothie recipe allows you to get your oatmeal fix without the usual long cooking time. You can throw the oats right into the blender for that nutty oatmeal taste.

INGREDIENTS | SERVES 2

1 cup steel-cut oats
1 cup ice
1 cup frozen mixed berries
1 tablespoon freshly grated ginger
1 teaspoon granulated stevia (optional)

Combine all ingredients in a blender and blend until smooth. Serve immediately.

Vegetable Frittata

Spinach, zucchini, and onion give this Vegetable Frittata a mild flavor with a powerhouse of nutrients. If you want to kick the flavor up a notch, you can add red peppers or hot peppers to the vegetables.

INGREDIENTS | SERVES 2

1 teaspoon water
½ medium zucchini, chopped
½ medium yellow onion, peeled and chopped
1 cup spinach
6 large egg whites
1 tablespoon chopped fresh parsley
¼ teaspoon salt
⅛ teaspoon ground black pepper

1. Preheat oven to 350°F. While oven is preheating, heat a medium skillet over medium-high heat and add water to pan. Add zucchini and onion and cook until soft, about 5 minutes. Add spinach and cook until wilted, about 3 minutes.

2. Remove vegetable mixture from heat.

3. In a medium bowl, whisk together egg whites, parsley, salt, and pepper.

4. Spread out vegetable mixture in the bottom of an 8" × 8" pan. Pour egg mixture on top.

5. Bake 20 minutes or until eggs are cooked through.

Open-Faced Breakfast Sandwich

Make this breakfast sandwich even more filling by adding some low-carbohydrate vegetables like zucchini, broccoli, or spinach.

INGREDIENTS | SERVES 2

4 slices turkey bacon
2 slices sprouted-grain bread
4 large egg whites
½ teaspoon salt
¼ teaspoon ground black pepper
1 teaspoon water

1. Heat a medium skillet over medium-high heat. When skillet is hot, add turkey bacon. Cook 3 minutes and then flip over. Cook another 3 minutes or until browned and cooked through. Set aside.

2. While bacon is cooking, toast sprouted-grain bread.

3. In a small bowl, whisk together eggs, salt, and pepper. Heat water in a medium skillet over medium heat and add egg mixture. Scramble until eggs are cooked through, about 3 minutes.

4. Put 2 slices turkey bacon on each toast slice and top each with half the egg mixture. Serve immediately.

Cinnamon Pumpkin Smoothie

For this recipe, you can use fresh or canned pumpkin purée. If you use canned, make sure you're purchasing 100 percent pumpkin purée and not pumpkin pie filling, which contains sugar and other undesirable ingredients.

INGREDIENTS | SERVES 2

1 cup pumpkin purée
1 cup water
¼ teaspoon ground cinnamon
¼ teaspoon vanilla extract
⅛ teaspoon ground ginger
1 teaspoon spirulina

Combine all ingredients in a blender and blend until smooth. Serve immediately.

Crazy Cinnamon

Cinnamon has the ability to imitate the activity of insulin in the body, which in turn helps control blood sugar levels. It also has the ability to alter the metabolism of carbohydrates so that they are more efficiently used as energy instead of stored as fat.

Turkey Fruit Salad

Many deli meats are cured with sugar or maple syrup. This recipe calls for sugar-free smoked turkey breast, so read your ingredient list before buying to make sure the turkey you're using is approved for Stage 1.

INGREDIENTS | SERVES 2

5 ounces smoked turkey breast (sugar-free), diced
1 cup cubed cantaloupe
1 cup cubed honeydew
½ cup sliced celery
1 teaspoon fresh lemon juice
1 tablespoon chopped scallions (green part only)

1. Combine turkey breast, cantaloupe, honeydew, and celery in a bowl. Toss with lemon juice. Sprinkle chopped scallions on top.

2. Refrigerate 30 minutes. Serve chilled.

Quinoa Breakfast Bowl

Quinoa is not just for dinner! This protein-packed pseudograin pairs nicely with eggs and smoked salmon.

INGREDIENTS | SERVES 2

½ cup quinoa, rinsed and drained

1 cup water

2 tablespoons chicken broth

2 tablespoons minced white onion

6 large egg whites

½ cup halved cherry tomatoes

4 ounces smoked salmon

The Power of Quinoa

Unlike wheat and rice, quinoa isn't technically a grain; it's more of a seed that's prepared and eaten like a grain. One-half cup of cooked quinoa contains 8 grams of protein, 5 grams of fiber, and 58 percent of the recommended daily allowance (RDA) for manganese—a mineral that's important for proper functioning of the thyroid gland.

1. Mix quinoa and water in a small saucepan and bring to a boil over high heat. Once water is boiling, reduce heat to low, cover, and allow to simmer 20 minutes or until quinoa is tender. Remove from heat and let stand 5 minutes.

2. Heat broth in a medium skillet over medium-high heat. Add onion and cook until translucent, about 5 minutes. Add egg whites and scramble until cooked through.

3. Add tomatoes and salmon and heat through. Transfer quinoa to skillet and toss to combine. Serve immediately.

Strawberry Pineapple Smoothie

You may use frozen fruit in place of fresh fruit for this smoothie, but you may have to increase the liquid if you do. Add a little splash of lemon juice in addition to some more water to really boost the flavor.

INGREDIENTS | SERVES 2

½ cup fresh whole strawberries, hulled
½ cup cubed fresh pineapple
2 tablespoons fresh lime juice
1 cup ice cubes
1 cup water
⅛ teaspoon freshly grated ginger

Combine all ingredients in a blender and blend until smooth.

Ginger the Great!

Ginger is widely known for its ability to reduce stomach upset, but ginger also helps balance blood sugar levels and may boost weight loss. The root has a strong, spicy flavor, so keep in mind that a little goes a long way.

Egg White Breakfast Burrito

This is a basic breakfast burrito recipe that you can make your own by adding any vegetables you want.

INGREDIENTS | SERVES 1

1 tablespoon water
1 tablespoon minced red pepper
1 tablespoon minced green pepper
1 tablespoon minced yellow pepper
1 tablespoon minced red onion
4 large egg whites
1 slice cooked turkey bacon, chopped
½ teaspoon salt
¼ teaspoon ground black pepper
1 sprouted-grain tortilla

1. Heat water in a medium skillet over medium-high heat. Add peppers and onion and cook until soft, about 5 minutes.

2. Whisk egg whites in a medium bowl and then add to onion and pepper mixture. Start scrambling. Once eggs start to cook, add turkey bacon, salt, and pepper. Continue cooking until eggs are set, about 3–4 minutes.

3. Remove from heat, transfer to tortilla, and roll tortilla up like a burrito. Serve immediately.

Egg White "Muffins"

One of the great things about these breakfast "muffins" is that you can prepare a dozen in advance and take them with you for breakfast on the go.

INGREDIENTS | SERVES 6

2 cups egg whites (about 24 egg whites)

2 cups baby spinach

1 medium red bell pepper, seeded and diced

½ cup chopped white mushrooms

½ teaspoon salt

¼ teaspoon ground black pepper

1. Preheat oven to 350°F.

2. Line each well of a twelve-cup muffin tin with a cupcake liner.

3. Whisk all ingredients together in a medium bowl and pour egg mixture evenly into each muffin tin. Bake 20–25 minutes or until egg is set.

CHAPTER 3

MD Stage 1 Lunch

Taco Bowls

In Stage 1 of this program, you can skip the rice and build your tacos on sprouted-grain or brown rice tortillas if you prefer.

INGREDIENTS | SERVES 2

1 cup brown rice

1½ cups water

½ pound lean ground beef

1 cup canned black beans, drained and rinsed

2 teaspoons taco seasoning (see Slow Cooker Cilantro Lime Chicken recipe in Chapter 4 for seasoning mix)

½ cup shredded lettuce

¼ cup salsa (no sugar added)

Choosing a Salsa

Many commercial salsas contain added sugar, so make sure you're checking the ingredient list. Natural sugar is okay, but avoid salsas that contain sugar, corn syrup, rice syrup, sucrose, dextrose, or any one of the other names for added sugar. Better yet, make your own!

1. Combine rice and water in a medium saucepan and bring to a boil. Once the mixture starts boiling, reduce heat to low, cover, and allow to simmer 20 minutes or until all water has been absorbed.

2. While rice is cooking, heat a medium skillet over medium heat. When skillet is hot, add ground beef and cook until no longer pink. Once meat is cooked, add beans and stir until beans are warm. Add taco seasoning and mix until combined.

3. Divide rice evenly between two bowls and then top each bowl with half the beef and bean mixture.

4. Top each bowl with ¼ cup shredded lettuce and ⅛ cup salsa.

Open-Faced Turkey Sandwich

Figs are one of the most perishable fruits, so they should only be purchased a day or two in advance of when you're planning to use them. Choose a fig that is rich in color and tender to the touch, but not mushy.

INGREDIENTS | SERVES 2

2 slices sprouted-grain bread

2 teaspoons yellow mustard

1 medium fresh fig

½ cup baby spinach

6 ounces roasted turkey breast, sliced

1. Toast sprouted bread. Spread each slice with 1 teaspoon yellow mustard.

2. Cut fig in half lengthwise and scoop out insides with a spoon. Spread half the fig on each bread slice. Top each slice with ¼ cup baby spinach and 3 ounces turkey breast.

Fiber in Figs

Figs are a good source of dietary fiber, containing about 1.5 grams per fig. Eating fiber-rich foods as part of your daily diet has a positive effect, not only on weight loss, but on long-term weight management.

Massaged Kale and Apple Salad

Massaging the kale for a few minutes with the lemon juice and salt helps make it soft and easier to eat. If you want to skip this step, or you prefer a softer "lettuce," choose baby kale.

INGREDIENTS | SERVES 2

4 cups kale

Juice from 1 medium lemon

¼ teaspoon sea salt

½ medium cucumber, diced

1 medium Granny Smith apple, cored and diced

2 tablespoons minced red onion

½ cup canned chickpeas, drained and rinsed

2 tablespoons balsamic vinegar

¼ teaspoon freshly ground black pepper

1. In a large bowl, combine kale, lemon juice, and sea salt. Massage ingredients together until kale starts to wilt, about 3 minutes.

2. Add cucumber, apple, onion, chickpeas, vinegar, and pepper and toss to combine.

3. Divide evenly into two serving bowls. Serve immediately.

Hearty Lentil Soup

There are several varieties of lentils available. The "regular" lentil that you'll typically encounter, especially in bulk sections of the grocery store, is the brown lentil or brewer lentil, but you can use any variety you find. They all have similar lentil-to-liquid ratios and cooking times.

INGREDIENTS | SERVES 4

2 teaspoons plus 2 cups water

1 small yellow onion, peeled and diced

2 stalks celery, diced

2 medium carrots, peeled and diced

2 cloves garlic, minced

4 cups vegetable broth

1 cup dried lentils, rinsed and drained

½ teaspoon salt

½ teaspoon ground black pepper

1 teaspoon Italian seasoning

½ cup chopped spinach

More for Your Money!

Who says that healthy eating has to be expensive? A cup of lentils runs about 20–30 cents and can supply one-third of the daily protein requirement for a 150-pound male. Lentils also help promote weight loss, stabilize blood sugar, and improve digestive health.

1. In a large stockpot, heat 2 teaspoons water over medium heat. Once hot, add onion, celery, and carrots and cook until soft, about 5 minutes. Add garlic and cook until fragrant, about 3 minutes.

2. Add broth, remaining water, and lentils and stir until combined. Turn heat to low and allow to simmer.

3. Once simmering, add salt, pepper, and Italian seasoning. Allow to simmer until lentils are soft, about 30–45 minutes.

4. Once lentils are soft, purée half the soup with an immersion blender or transfer to a regular blender. Stir in puréed soup with nonpuréed soup and add spinach. Serve warm.

Brown Rice Stir-Fry

This is a basic stir-fry that you can adjust to your own tastes. Switch up the vegetables or use different meats. You can even swap the brown rice for wild long-grain rice, if you prefer it.

INGREDIENTS | SERVES 2

1 cup brown rice

1½ cups water

2 tablespoons coconut aminos

1 small yellow onion, peeled and minced

½ medium red bell pepper, seeded and diced

½ medium green bell pepper, seeded and diced

1 medium zucchini, diced

6 ounces boneless skinless chicken breast, cut into 1" cubes

1 teaspoon hot sauce

¼ teaspoon salt

⅛ teaspoon ground black pepper

½ cup pea shoots

Pick Those Pea Shoots!

Pea shoots are sprouted peas that are loaded with nutrition. One cup provides about 35 percent of your daily vitamin C needs and 15 percent of your daily vitamin A needs. They are also an excellent source of vitamin K, providing 66 percent of your needs for the day.

1. In a small saucepan, combine rice and water over high heat. Bring to a boil and then reduce heat to low and cover. Allow to simmer until rice is soft, about 20 minutes.

2. Put coconut aminos in a wok or large skillet over medium heat. Add onion and cook until translucent, about 5 minutes. Add peppers and cook until soft, about 5 more minutes. Add zucchini and cook until soft but still slightly crisp.

3. Add chicken and cook until no longer pink, about 10 minutes. Stir in hot sauce, salt, and pepper.

4. Remove from heat. Divide rice evenly into two bowls and top each bowl with half the stir-fry mixture. Top each bowl with ¼ cup pea shoots. Serve warm.

Savory Bacon and Chive Oatmeal

The word "oatmeal" usually conjures up images of brown sugar, maple syrup, raisins, or some other sweet concoction, but don't let that scare you away from this savory version of the hearty breakfast staple. You may never go back.

INGREDIENTS | SERVES 2

4 slices sugar-free turkey bacon

1½ cups chicken stock

½ cup water

½ cup steel-cut oats

2 tablespoons chopped fresh chives, plus 1 tablespoon for garnish

¼ teaspoon salt

¼ teaspoon ground black pepper

1. Heat a medium skillet over medium-high heat. Put bacon in skillet and cook until browned and crispy, about 4–5 minutes on each side. Remove bacon from heat and set aside.

2. Combine stock and water in a medium saucepan and bring to a slow boil over high heat. Stir in steel-cut oats and reduce heat to low.

3. Allow to simmer 20–25 minutes or until liquid is absorbed, stirring occasionally.

4. While oats are cooking, roughly chop bacon. Once liquid is absorbed, stir in bacon bits, 2 tablespoons chives, salt, and pepper. Garnish with remaining 1 tablespoon chives. Serve warm.

Lemon Shrimp with Brown Rice Linguini

This recipe calls for brown rice linguini, but you can use any brown rice variety you'd like such as spaghetti, ziti, or penne.

INGREDIENTS | SERVES 4

6 cups water

8 ounces brown rice linguini

½ cup chicken broth

¼ cup white wine vinegar

Juice from 1 large lemon

¼ teaspoon salt

¼ teaspoon ground black pepper

⅛ teaspoon lemon pepper

1 pound raw medium shrimp, peeled and deveined

¼ cup chopped parsley

Don't Overcook

Brown rice pasta tends to get soft faster than traditional wheat pasta. Keep an eye on your pasta while it's cooking, testing it as you go. Remove it from the water when it's the right texture for you.

1. Bring water to a boil in a large stockpot over high heat. Add brown rice linguini and cook until al dente, about 7 minutes. Drain and set aside.

2. In a large skillet, combine broth, vinegar, and lemon juice over medium heat. Bring to a boil, uncovered, and allow to boil until the sauce thickens and is reduced by half, about 10 minutes.

3. Add salt, black pepper, and lemon pepper and stir until combined. Cook 1 more minute.

4. Add shrimp and cook until pink, about 3 minutes. Pour shrimp and sauce mixture over brown rice linguini. Top with parsley. Serve immediately.

Three-Bean Chili

This recipe has some kick. If you'd rather dial back the spice, you can omit the chili powder or swap the fire-roasted diced tomatoes for regular diced tomatoes.

INGREDIENTS | SERVES 8

4 cups vegetable broth

1 small yellow onion, peeled and diced

1 large red pepper, seeded and diced

1 small jalapeño pepper, seeded and diced

1 (15-ounce) can black beans, drained and rinsed

1 (15-ounce) can red kidney beans, drained and rinsed

1 (15-ounce) can white cannellini beans, drained and rinsed

1 cup dried lentils, rinsed and drained

1 (15-ounce) can crushed tomatoes

1 (15-ounce) can fire-roasted diced tomatoes

1 tablespoon chili powder

1 teaspoon ground cumin

½ teaspoon garlic powder

½ teaspoon onion powder

½ teaspoon salt

¼ teaspoon ground black pepper

¼ cup chopped fresh cilantro

1. Mix all ingredients, except the cilantro, in a slow cooker and cook on low 8–10 hours or 4–6 hours on high.

2. Serve warm garnished with cilantro if desired.

More Than a Garnish

Cilantro is often brushed off as a garnish, but this green not only enhances the flavor of black beans, it has powerful nutritional benefits too. Cilantro is a natural cleansing agent—it helps cleanse the blood of toxic metals by binding to them and removing them from body tissue.

Sprouted Tuna Wrap

For Stage 1, it's important to choose tuna that's packed in water instead of oil. Most popular tuna companies have both options readily available at the store, so pay attention to the labels as you shop.

INGREDIENTS | SERVES 2

1 (5-ounce) can tuna packed in water

2 hard-boiled large eggs, peeled, yolks removed, and whites chopped

2 teaspoons yellow mustard

1 tablespoon minced white onion

¼ teaspoon seasoned salt

¼ teaspoon ground black pepper

2 sprouted-grain tortillas

½ cup pea shoots

1. In a medium bowl, mix together tuna, chopped egg whites, mustard, onion, seasoned salt, and pepper until combined.

2. Add tuna mixture evenly to each tortilla and top with ¼ cup pea shoots each. Roll tortillas and secure with a toothpick. Serve immediately.

Mustard-Roasted Salmon

If you can, choose wild Alaskan salmon for this recipe. Farmed salmon is often injected with chemicals that make the fish's flesh appear pinker.

INGREDIENTS | SERVES 2

2 (6-ounce) salmon fillets

3 tablespoons spicy mustard

1 teaspoon white vinegar

½ teaspoon salt

½ teaspoon ground black pepper

1 tablespoon minced shallots

1. Preheat oven to 400°F. Line a baking sheet with parchment paper and place salmon fillets on top.

2. In a small bowl, whisk together mustard, vinegar, salt, pepper, and shallots.

3. Spread the mustard mixture equally in a thin layer over each fillet.

4. Bake salmon 15–20 minutes or until fish flakes easily. Serve immediately.

Sweet Potato and Black Bean Burrito

You can adapt this vegetarian recipe to appeal to the meat lover by adding some lean ground turkey or cubed chicken breasts to the mix.

INGREDIENTS | SERVES 4

2 medium sweet potatoes, peeled and diced

½ teaspoon ground cinnamon

¼ teaspoon coarse sea salt

1 (15-ounce) can black beans, drained and rinsed

½ teaspoon ground cumin

¼ teaspoon garlic powder

¼ teaspoon onion powder

⅛ teaspoon cayenne pepper

4 sprouted-grain tortillas

½ teaspoon hot sauce (no sugar added)

The Power of Cayenne

The cayenne pepper in hot sauce doesn't just give your food some bite; it actually can help boost metabolism and speed weight loss.

1. Preheat oven to 400°F. Line a baking sheet with parchment paper and set aside.

2. In a medium bowl, toss sweet potatoes with cinnamon and coarse sea salt. Spread potatoes out on baking sheet. Bake 20–25 minutes (turning once while baking) or until sweet potatoes are crisp and soft.

3. While potatoes are cooking, heat a small skillet over medium heat. Put beans in skillet and add cumin, garlic powder, onion powder, and cayenne. Cook until beans are warm and spices are combined, about 6 minutes. Remove from heat.

4. When potatoes are done cooking, combine potatoes and beans in a medium bowl. Divide mixture evenly between each tortilla and top with hot sauce if desired. Roll burrito and secure with a toothpick. Serve immediately.

Lemon Chicken Breast

This lemon pepper spice mixture also goes well with any type of whitefish, so you can swap the chicken breasts out for your favorite aquatic variety if you're looking for a somewhat leaner option.

INGREDIENTS | SERVES 2

½ teaspoon salt

½ teaspoon ground black pepper

½ teaspoon lemon pepper

¼ teaspoon smoked paprika

¼ teaspoon dried parsley

2 (4-ounce) boneless skinless chicken breasts

2 tablespoons chicken broth

1 large lemon

2 teaspoons chopped fresh parsley

Sprinkle on the Paprika

Paprika belongs to the *Capsicum annuum* (red pepper) species, which also includes cayenne and red pepper flakes. The capsaicin in paprika can help rev up metabolism and make you feel fuller longer.

1. Combine salt, black pepper, lemon pepper, paprika, and parsley in a gallon-sized plastic bag. Shake to mix well. Place chicken breasts in bag and shake to coat with spice mixture.

2. Heat broth in a large skillet over medium heat. Add chicken breasts and cook 5 minutes on each side or until no longer pink. When chicken is almost done cooking, squeeze juice from lemon on each breast.

3. Remove from heat and top with fresh parsley. Serve immediately.

Sardine Salad

You can top this salad with any kind of protein you like. Swap the sardines for tuna, salmon, chicken, or even crabmeat. Make it vegetarian by adding some chickpeas or beans.

INGREDIENTS | SERVES 2

4 cups mixed greens

Juice from 1 medium lemon

3 tablespoons balsamic vinegar (no sugar added)

½ teaspoon salt

¼ teaspoon ground black pepper

¼ cup chopped beets

½ cup chopped tomatoes

½ cup chopped celery

1 (4.3-ounce) can sardines, packed in water

1. In a large bowl, combine mixed greens, lemon juice, vinegar, salt, and pepper. Toss to mix well. Top with beets, tomatoes, and celery and toss again.

2. Chop sardines and place on top of salad. Serve immediately.

The Sunshine Vitamin D

Very few foods naturally contain vitamin D—sardines are one of those foods. Just one can of sardines gets you 63 percent of your daily dose of vitamin D and over 100 percent of your vitamin B_{12}.

Turkey Meatloaf

Forget the bread crumbs. The steel-cut oats in this recipe help hold the meatloaf together while also keeping it moist and delicious.

INGREDIENTS | SERVES 4

2 tablespoons chicken broth
1 cup chopped white onion
3 cloves garlic, minced
1 pound ground turkey
¼ cup steel-cut oats
2 large egg whites
¾ cup ketchup (sugar-free), divided
2 teaspoons coconut aminos
½ teaspoon salt
½ teaspoon ground black pepper

1. Preheat oven to 350°F.

2. Heat broth in a medium skillet over medium heat. Add onion and garlic and cook until translucent, about 5 minutes. Remove from heat and set aside.

3. In a large bowl, combine turkey, oats, egg whites, ¼ cup ketchup, coconut aminos, salt, and pepper. Add onion and garlic mixture. Mix well.

4. Place turkey mixture in a loaf pan and cover with remaining ½ cup ketchup.

5. Bake 50 minutes or until a meat thermometer reads 165°F. Allow to cool 5 minutes before serving.

Quinoa Summer Squash Salad

This summer salad is the perfect side dish for your next outdoor barbecue. It's loaded with protein, vitamins, and minerals and is always a crowd pleaser.

INGREDIENTS | SERVES 4

½ cup quinoa, rinsed and drained
1 cup vegetable or chicken broth
2 medium zucchini, diced
2 medium yellow squash, diced
½ teaspoon salt
½ teaspoon ground black pepper
½ teaspoon ground sage

1. Preheat oven to 375°F. Line a baking sheet with parchment paper.

2. In a medium saucepan, combine quinoa and broth over high heat. Stir until combined and allow to come to a boil. Boil 1 minute, then cover and reduce heat to low. Allow to simmer 20 minutes or until quinoa is soft.

3. While quinoa is cooking, toss zucchini and yellow squash with salt, pepper, and sage in a medium bowl. Spread out mixture on the baking sheet and cook 20 minutes or until vegetables are browned and soft. Remove from oven and toss with quinoa.

4. Serve immediately.

Sun-Dried Tomato, Kale, and Bean Salad

Instead of canned beans, you can use dried beans in this recipe. If you decide to use dried beans, you'll need to prepare in advance by soaking the beans for at least 8 hours to overnight.

INGREDIENTS | SERVES 2

2 cups roughly chopped kale

1 tablespoon lime juice

1 tablespoon lemon juice

½ cup canned black beans, drained and rinsed

½ cup canned white beans, drained and rinsed

½ cup canned kidney beans, drained and rinsed

¼ cup diced celery

¼ teaspoon salt

¼ teaspoon ground black pepper

1. In a medium bowl, add kale and drizzle with lime and lemon juice. Massage kale until it starts to soften, about 1–2 minutes.

2. Add remaining ingredients and toss to coat. Refrigerate 30 minutes. Serve chilled.

Beans, Beans—They're Good for Your Heart

Beans contain phytochemicals—naturally occurring compounds found in plants—that can protect against heart disease. They're also full of isoflavones and phytosterols, which are associated with a reduced risk of cancer.

Salmon Salad Sandwich

The combination of apple cider vinegar and lemon juice make this salmon salad nice and tangy. When choosing a canned salmon, make sure it's wild-caught.

INGREDIENTS | SERVES 2

1 (6-ounce) can wild Alaskan salmon

2 tablespoons minced red onion

2 tablespoons lemon juice

1 teaspoon apple cider vinegar

¼ teaspoon ground black pepper

4 slices sprouted-grain bread

2 tablespoons hummus

4 slices tomato

4 leaves romaine lettuce

1. In a small bowl, combine salmon, onion, lemon juice, vinegar, and pepper. Set aside.

2. Toast each bread slice and spread each with ½ tablespoon hummus.

3. Top 2 bread slices with 2 slices tomato, 2 lettuce leaves, and half the salmon mixture. Cover with remaining bread. Serve immediately.

Brain Food

Salmon is often referred to as "brain food" because it's rich in omega-3 fatty acids—a type of fat that is essential in infant brain development and reduces the risk of mental disorders like depression and Alzheimer's disease.

Curried Red Lentil Soup

*Don't let the jalapeño scare you away from this recipe—it gives just
the right amount of kick without being too spicy.*

INGREDIENTS | SERVES 6

1 tablespoon water

1 large yellow onion, peeled and diced

2 cloves garlic, minced

1 tablespoon minced fresh ginger

1 medium jalapeño pepper, seeded and minced

1 tablespoon curry powder

1½ teaspoons ground cumin

½ teaspoon ground turmeric

1 teaspoon ground cinnamon

1½ cups dried red lentils, rinsed and drained

8 cups chicken broth

½ tablespoon dried parsley

2 tablespoons lemon juice

1 teaspoon salt

½ teaspoon ground black pepper

2 tablespoons fresh-chopped parsley

1. Heat water in a large stockpot over medium heat. Add onion and garlic and cook until translucent, about 3–4 minutes.

2. Add ginger, jalapeño, curry, cumin, turmeric, and cinnamon and cook until fragrant, about 3 minutes.

3. Add lentils and broth and bring to a boil. Reduce heat to low and stir in dried parsley, lemon juice, salt, and pepper. Allow to simmer 45–60 minutes or until lentils are soft.

4. Garnish with fresh parsley.

Chicken and Vegetable Soup

*Make sure you're adding uncooked rice to this recipe. As the soup simmers,
the rice will absorb enough of the broth to make it tender.*

INGREDIENTS | SERVES 2

2 tablespoons water

8 ounces boneless skinless chicken breasts, cut into cubes

1 small zucchini, diced

2 medium carrots, peeled and chopped

1 medium shallot, peeled and diced

2 medium Roma tomatoes, diced

1½ cups baby spinach

1 (14-ounce) can chicken broth

2 tablespoons uncooked brown rice

½ teaspoon Italian seasoning

¼ teaspoon dried thyme

¼ teaspoon salt

¼ teaspoon ground black pepper

1. Heat water in a medium skillet over medium heat and add cubed chicken. Cook until browned and no longer pink, about 6–8 minutes. Remove from pan with a slotted spoon.

2. Add zucchini, carrots, and shallot to pan and cook over medium heat until soft, about 4 minutes. Add tomatoes and cook until just heated through, about 2 minutes.

3. Transfer vegetable mixture and chicken to a large stockpot or large saucepan and add remaining ingredients.

4. Bring to a boil over high heat and then reduce heat to low and allow to simmer 20 minutes.

Brown versus White

Unlike white rice, brown rice still contains two components of the grain—the bran and the hull—that are rich in protein, thiamine, calcium, magnesium, and fiber. Brown rice also has a lower glycemic index, so it won't affect blood sugar and insulin levels as much as white rice.

Chicken and Apple Salad

*As this chicken and apple salad sits, it tends to develop more flavor. Prepare
the salad in advance the night before (and store in the refrigerator), and
then scoop it over mixed greens when you're ready to serve.*

INGREDIENTS | SERVES 4

1 (12.5-ounce) can shredded
chicken breast

1 medium Granny Smith apple, cored
and chopped

1 celery stalk, diced

2 tablespoons minced white onion

3 tablespoons chopped sun-
dried tomatoes

1 tablespoon lemon juice

1 teaspoon apple cider vinegar

¼ teaspoon seasoned salt

¼ teaspoon ground black pepper

4 cups mixed greens

Mix all ingredients except mixed greens together in a
medium bowl until combined. Serve over mixed greens.

CHAPTER 4

MD Stage 1 Dinner

Shrimp Skewers with Mango Salsa

If you're using wooden skewers, allow them to soak in water for at least an hour before grilling with them. This will reduce the risk of them catching on fire.

INGREDIENTS | SERVES 2

1 small mango, peeled and cubed

1 green onion, chopped

3 tablespoons minced red onion

2 tablespoons chopped cilantro

1 small jalapeño pepper, seeded and minced

Juice from 1 large lime plus 2 tablespoons

⅛ teaspoon plus ½ teaspoon salt

2 tablespoons smoked paprika

½ teaspoon ground cumin

1 teaspoon minced garlic

½ teaspoon ground black pepper

1 pound raw large shrimp, peeled and deveined

1. Mix mango, green onion, red onion, cilantro, jalapeño, juice from 1 lime, and ⅛ teaspoon salt in a large bowl. Cover and allow to chill at least 30 minutes.

2. While salsa is chilling, preheat the grill. Combine paprika, cumin, garlic, remaining salt, pepper, and 2 tablespoons lime juice in a shallow baking dish. Form kebabs by dividing shrimp evenly between the skewers. Place shrimp kebabs in marinade and allow to chill 30 minutes in the refrigerator.

3. Grill shrimp kebabs 2–4 minutes on each side or until shrimp is completely pink.

4. Remove from grill, top with mango salsa, and serve immediately.

Beauty Food

Shrimp are sometimes referred to as a "beauty food" because they contain astaxanthin—the carotenoid that protects against premature aging of the skin. This carotenoid also gives them their pink color.

Pulled Pork with Sweet Potatoes

This recipe requires some preparation as it's best to season the pork and allow it to sit in the refrigerator overnight to fully develop its flavor. It's well worth the wait.

INGREDIENTS | SERVES 4

1 teaspoon chili powder

1 teaspoon ground cumin

1½ teaspoons smoked paprika

1 teaspoon ground black pepper

1 teaspoon salt

½ teaspoon dried oregano

¼ teaspoon cayenne pepper (optional)

1 (1-pound) pork tenderloin

¼ cup water

2 medium white onions, peeled and cut into rings

2 medium Gala apples, peeled, cored, and cubed

2 medium sweet potatoes, peeled and cubed

1. In a small bowl, combine chili powder, cumin, paprika, pepper, salt, oregano, and cayenne. Rub spice mixture over pork loin, making sure to get it in all the creases and crevices. Wrap pork loin in plastic wrap and refrigerate overnight.

2. Pour water in slow cooker and line bottom of slow cooker with onions. Put pork on top of onions and then apples and sweet potatoes on top of pork.

3. Cook in slower cooker on low 6 hours. Shred pork with a fork and mix with apple-potato mixture before serving.

Slow Cooker Cilantro Lime Chicken

Most taco seasoning packets are full of additives like MSG, sugar, and cornstarch. It's simple—and much more delicious—to make your own with spices that you probably already have on hand.

INGREDIENTS | SERVES 4

1 tablespoon chili powder

¼ teaspoon garlic powder

¼ teaspoon onion powder

¼ teaspoon dried oregano

½ teaspoon paprika

1 teaspoon ground cumin

1 teaspoon salt

1 teaspoon ground black pepper

4 (4-ounce) boneless skinless chicken breasts

1 small white onion, peeled and cubed

2 cloves garlic, minced

1 (15.5-ounce) can black beans, drained and rinsed

2 medium limes

1 (16-ounce) jar salsa (no sugar added)

¼ cup chopped cilantro

1. Mix spices together in a large plastic bag. Put chicken breasts in plastic bag and shake to coat.

2. Line bottom of a slow cooker with onion, garlic, and beans. Put chicken breasts on top of beans and squeeze lime juice over them. Pour salsa on top.

3. Cook on low 6–8 hours or until chicken is moist and tender. Top with cilantro before serving.

Cuminaldehyde in Cumin

One of the major health benefits of cumin is its ability to aid in digestion. Just the smell of cumin, which comes from a compound called cuminaldehyde, activates the salivary glands, which start the digestive process.

Seared Scallop Salad

This recipe calls for sea scallops, which are large in size. You can replace the sea scallops with bay scallops—a smaller variety—but if you do, you may want to increase the quantity.

INGREDIENTS | SERVES 4

1 tablespoon lemon pepper

1 teaspoon salt

2 teaspoons ground black pepper, divided

20 large sea scallops

8 cups mixed greens

1 cup chopped grape tomatoes

¼ cup chopped red onion

1 medium cucumber, sliced

⅓ cup mustard

¼ cup raw apple cider vinegar

1 tablespoon water

1. Preheat grill to medium-high heat.

2. Combine lemon pepper, salt, and 1 teaspoon pepper in a large bowl. Place scallops in bowl and toss to coat.

3. Grill scallops 2–3 minutes on each side or until cooked through.

4. In a large bowl, mix together greens, tomatoes, onion, and cucumber.

5. In a separate small bowl, whisk together mustard, vinegar, water, and remaining 1 teaspoon pepper. Pour dressing over greens and toss to coat.

6. Top with scallops. Serve immediately.

Spaghetti and Meat Sauce

This recipe is pure comfort food—it will give your grandmother's spaghetti and meatballs a run for their money.

INGREDIENTS | SERVES 6

1 pound lean ground beef

½ pound hot Italian pork sausage (no sugar added), casings removed

4 (8-ounce) cans tomato sauce (no sugar added)

2 (6-ounce) cans tomato paste (no sugar added)

2 cloves garlic, minced

2 teaspoons Italian seasoning

1 teaspoon salt

½ teaspoon ground black pepper

½ teaspoon red pepper flakes

6 cups water

1 pound brown rice spaghetti

½ cup chopped fresh parsley

1. In a large stockpot, cook ground beef and Italian sausage over medium-high heat until no longer pink. Drain excess fat.

2. Add tomato sauce, tomato paste, garlic, Italian seasoning, salt, black pepper, and red pepper flakes and bring to a boil over medium-high heat. Boil 1 minute then reduce heat to low. Allow to simmer uncovered 1 hour, stirring occasionally.

3. In another large pot, bring water to a boil over high heat. Add brown rice spaghetti. Cook uncovered 6–8 minutes or until spaghetti reaches desired doneness. Drain pasta and add to serving bowl.

4. Pour sauce over spaghetti. Garnish with fresh parsley.

Reading Sausage Labels

Many commercial sausages are made with some type of sugar or corn syrup. When using sausage, you must read your labels diligently to avoid these added ingredients. It's usually best to visit your local farmer or butcher to find sausages that are fresh and additive-free. If you can't find sausage without added sugar, you can use ground pork instead.

Chicken Taco Soup

Simmering this soup in a slow cooker for a few hours really allows the flavors to develop, but if you're in a rush to get dinner on the table, you can prepare this soup in a stockpot and serve once it's heated through.

INGREDIENTS | SERVES 6

1 (15.5-ounce) can black beans, drained and rinsed

1 (15.5-ounce) can pinto beans, drained and rinsed

1 (14.5-ounce) can fire-roasted diced tomatoes

1 (12.5-ounce) can chicken breast in water

1 (15-ounce) can low-fat refried beans

1 (14-ounce) can chicken broth

1 tablespoon chili powder

¼ teaspoon garlic powder

¼ teaspoon onion powder

¼ teaspoon dried oregano

½ teaspoon paprika

1 teaspoon ground cumin

1 teaspoon salt

1 teaspoon ground black pepper

1 (4-ounce) can green chilies

1. Combine all ingredients in a slow cooker. Stir until seasonings dissolve.

2. Cook on low heat 3 hours.

Protein Power

Refried beans are a staple of Mexican and Tex-Mex cuisine. They are made by boiling and frying pinto beans in advance, mashing them, and heating when ready to use. A single cup of refried beans contains 13 grams of protein and 12 grams of fiber.

Slow Cooker Adobo Chicken

Adobo refers to a cooking process in Philippine cuisine that involves marinating meat, seafood, or vegetables in a combination of vinegar, soy sauce, and garlic. Soy is out for all stages, but coconut aminos make a more than suitable replacement.

INGREDIENTS | SERVES 8

1 small sweet onion, peeled and chopped roughly

¾ cup coconut aminos

¼ cup red wine vinegar

1 teaspoon ground ginger

6 cloves garlic, crushed

1 teaspoon whole black peppercorns

2 bay leaves

1 (4-pound) whole chicken

1. In a small bowl, combine onion, coconut aminos, vinegar, ginger, garlic, peppercorns, and bay leaves.

2. Put chicken in slow cooker and pour mixture over chicken. Cook on low 6–8 hours or until chicken is cooked through.

Pepper for Digestion

Black pepper stimulates the taste buds, which signals the stomach to increase production of hydrochloric acid (HCl). HCl is necessary for proper digestion, mainly of protein.

Cilantro Lime Chickpea Salad

If you prefer to cook your own chickpeas (also called garbanzo beans) instead of using a canned variety, rinse and then presoak them in a saucepan with 3 cups of water per 1 cup of beans. Boil for 2 minutes, remove from heat, and then allow to sit for 4 hours.

INGREDIENTS | SERVES 2

1 clove garlic, crushed

2 teaspoons spicy mustard

Juice from 1 medium lime

½ teaspoon salt

½ teaspoon ground black pepper

1 (15.5-ounce) can chickpeas, drained and rinsed

1 (15.5-ounce) can cannellini beans, drained and rinsed

2 cups roughly chopped spinach

½ cup chopped cilantro

¼ cup chopped white onion

1. Add garlic, mustard, lime juice, salt, and pepper to a small bowl and mix thoroughly.

2. In a large bowl, combine chickpeas, cannellini beans, spinach, cilantro, and onion.

3. Add mustard and lime mixture to chickpea mixture and toss to coat. Refrigerate 30–60 minutes. Serve chilled.

Heart-Healthy Chickpeas

Just 2 cups of garbanzo beans supply almost all the fiber you need in an entire day. The fiber in these beans, along with the other nutrients they contain, helps regulate blood sugar levels and can lower the blood lipids that increase your risk for heart disease.

Sloppy Joes

Typically, sloppy Joes contain added sugar, but you won't even miss it when you try this recipe. Like most tomato-based dishes, this recipe tastes better after sitting for a day or two. Serve over lettuce leaves.

INGREDIENTS | SERVES 8

2 tablespoons chicken broth

1 medium yellow onion, peeled and chopped

2 cloves garlic, minced

1 medium red bell pepper, seeded and diced

2 pounds lean ground beef

2 (14.5-ounce) cans diced tomato

1 (6-ounce) can tomato paste

1 cup sliced mushrooms

2 tablespoons coconut aminos

2 teaspoons chili powder

½ teaspoon salt

½ teaspoon ground black pepper

1. Heat broth in a large skillet over medium-high heat. Add onion and garlic and cook until translucent, about 4–5 minutes. Add red pepper and continue to cook for another 5 minutes or until pepper is tender. Add beef and cook until no longer pink, about 6–7 minutes.

2. Transfer meat mixture to a slow cooker. Add remaining ingredients and cook on low 4–6 hours.

Garlic Pork Roast

Pork shoulder (also called pork butt) is a tough cut that's layered with fat so it's good for slow cooking because it tends to stay moister than other cuts. When you shred the pork, you'll be able to remove any excess fat.

INGREDIENTS | SERVES 4

1 (2-pound) boneless pork shoulder

2 teaspoons salt

2 teaspoons ground black pepper

5 cloves garlic, thinly sliced

1 medium yellow onion, peeled and chopped

2 medium carrots, peeled and chopped

2 stalks celery, chopped

1½ cups chicken broth

1. Rub pork shoulder with salt and pepper. Make small incisions in the pork shoulder with a paring knife. Stuff a garlic piece in each slice.

2. Put pork roast in a slow cooker and cover with onion, carrots, and celery. Pour broth on top.

3. Cook on low 6 hours or until pork comes apart easily with a fork.

Pork Butt?

Although pork shoulder is also referred to as pork butt, it doesn't actually come from the pork's rear end. In this case, the word "butt" refers to the old English term for "the widest part." On the pig, the widest part is the shoulder.

Pumpkin and Sweet Potato Chili

This chili combines hearty autumn vegetables and rich fall spices.
It's perfect for when the weather starts to cool down.

INGREDIENTS | SERVES 6

1 teaspoon salt

2 tablespoons chili powder

2 teaspoons ground cumin

1 teaspoon dried oregano

½ teaspoon ground cinnamon

1 teaspoon unsweetened cocoa powder

¼ teaspoon ground allspice

2 tablespoons chicken broth

1 small white onion, peeled and finely diced

2 cloves garlic, minced

1 pound lean ground beef

2 medium sweet potatoes, peeled and diced

1 (15-ounce) can pumpkin purée

1 (15.5-ounce) can fire-roasted diced tomatoes

2 cups beef broth

¼ cup chopped cilantro

1. Mix spices in a small bowl. Set aside.

2. Heat broth in a large stockpot over medium heat. Add onion and garlic and cook until translucent, about 5 minutes. Add beef and cook until no longer pink, about 6–7 minutes.

3. Add spice mixture to beef and stir until evenly incorporated.

4. Add remaining ingredients except cilantro and stir until combined. Simmer 1 hour.

5. Serve garnished with cilantro.

Powerful Pumpkin

The most well known use of pumpkin may be as a sugar-laden pie filling, but fall's signature squash packs a powerful nutritional punch. Pumpkin improves eyesight, reduces the risk of heart disease, and helps you keep your waistline in check.

Grilled Flank Steak

Flank steak is the long and flat meat cut from the abdominal muscles or butt of the cow. You can also use skirt steak, which is cut from a cow's diaphragm muscle, as a substitute for flank steak.

INGREDIENTS | SERVES 4

2 cloves garlic, minced
¼ cup balsamic vinegar
¼ cup coconut aminos
2 tablespoons spicy brown mustard
2 teaspoons dried rosemary
1 teaspoon dried thyme
1 teaspoon salt
½ teaspoon ground black pepper
1 (1-pound) flank steak

1. In a large mixing bowl, whisk garlic, vinegar, coconut aminos, mustard, rosemary, thyme, salt, and pepper.

2. Put flank steak in a large sealable plastic bag. Pour marinade over steak and seal bag, squeezing out excess air. Marinate in refrigerator 1 hour.

3. Heat up a grill to medium-high heat and place steak on grate. Cook 6–8 minutes on each side or until steak reaches desired doneness, brushing with marinade as it cooks.

4. Remove steak from heat and let stand 5 minutes before cutting.

Slow Cooker Lemon Garlic Chicken

If you're pressed for time, you can make this dish in the oven instead of the slow cooker. Follow the directions as written, but cook the chicken at 350°F for 35–40 minutes or until the juices run clear.

INGREDIENTS | SERVES 6

2 teaspoons dried oregano
2 teaspoons dried parsley
1 teaspoon seasoned salt
1 teaspoon ground black pepper
6 (4-ounce) boneless skinless chicken breasts
¼ cup chicken broth
¼ cup lemon juice
2 cloves garlic, minced

1. Combine oregano, parsley, salt, and pepper in a gallon-sized plastic bag. Put chicken breasts in the bag and shake until coated.

2. Place chicken breasts in the bottom of a slow cooker. Add broth, lemon juice, and garlic.

3. Cook on low 6 hours or until chicken comes apart easily with a fork.

Roasted Butternut Squash and Apple Soup

You can save yourself some time and a lot of effort by buying precubed butternut squash. Some grocery stores even carry frozen cubed butternut squash that works nicely with this recipe—just defrost first.

INGREDIENTS | SERVES 8

1 tablespoon chicken stock

1 medium yellow onion, peeled and chopped

8 cups cubed butternut squash

2 medium Granny Smith apples, peeled, cored, and cubed

½ medium red bell pepper, seeded and chopped

3 cloves garlic, chopped

8 cups chicken or vegetable broth

2 teaspoons salt

1. In a large stockpot, heat chicken stock over medium-high heat. Add onion and cook until translucent, about 5 minutes. Add squash, apples, bell pepper, garlic, broth, and salt.

2. Bring to a boil and then reduce heat to low and simmer 25–30 minutes or until squash is tender.

3. Transfer ingredients to a blender or use an immersion blender to purée.

4. Serve warm.

Butternut for Blood Sugar

Like other types of winter squash, butternut squash is particularly effective in helping to control blood sugar levels. The polysaccharides—or long-chain carbohydrates—in the squash's cell wall improve the regulation of insulin, which controls blood sugar.

Fish Tacos with Pineapple Salsa

Haddock is a member of the cod family, so it's subject to the same overfishing problems. When choosing haddock, opt for a certified sustainable fishery.

INGREDIENTS | SERVES 2

1 cup diced pineapple

¼ cup minced red onion

¼ cup chopped cilantro plus 2 tablespoons for garnish

1 small jalapeño pepper, seeded and minced

⅛ teaspoon plus ½ teaspoon salt

Juice from 1 medium lime

½ teaspoon onion powder

½ teaspoon garlic powder

½ teaspoon paprika

½ teaspoon ground black pepper

2 (6-ounce) haddock fillets

4 (6") sprouted-grain tortillas

1. Combine pineapple, red onion, ¼ cilantro, jalapeño, ⅛ teaspoon salt, and lime juice in a small bowl. Toss to combine and refrigerate for 1 hour.

2. Place an oven rack 6" from heat source and set oven to broil.

3. Mix onion powder, garlic powder, paprika, ½ teaspoon salt, and pepper together in a small bowl.

4. Line a baking sheet with foil and set haddock fillets flat on baking sheet. Sprinkle with seasoning mixture.

5. Broil 6 minutes or until fish flakes easily with a fork.

6. Top each tortilla with 3 ounces fish and a spoonful pineapple salsa. Garnish with remaining cilantro if desired.

Pork Chops with Fresh Applesauce

Homemade applesauce is a cinch to make and doesn't require more than four ingredients. If you prefer to buy, make sure to choose a bottled variety that doesn't contain any added sugar or artificial ingredients.

INGREDIENTS | SERVES 4

½ teaspoon dried thyme

½ teaspoon salt

½ teaspoon ground black pepper

4 (4-ounce) pork chops, trimmed of fat

2 tablespoons chicken broth

4 medium apples, peeled, cored, and diced

1 teaspoon ground cinnamon

⅛ teaspoon ground nutmeg

¾ cup water

2 slices lemon

Thyme to Get Healthy

Thyme isn't just a flavor booster; the herb is packed with vitamin C and is also a good source of vitamin A—two vitamins that boost your immune system and help you fight off infection.

1. In a small bowl, combine thyme, salt, and pepper. Rub the mixture over pork chops.

2. Heat a medium skillet over medium heat and put broth in pan. Add pork chops and cook 5–6 minutes per side or until browned and the inside is no longer pink. Set aside to rest, tented with foil to keep warm.

3. Add apples, cinnamon, nutmeg, water, and lemon to a medium saucepan. Bring to a boil over high heat, then cover and reduce heat to low. Simmer 20 minutes or until apples are completely soft, stirring frequently. Remove from heat and place in food processor. Pulse until smooth or until applesauce reaches desired consistency.

4. Top pork chops with applesauce. Serve warm.

Chicken Sausage with Brown Rice Pasta

Chicken sausage comes in many varieties from chicken and apple to sun-dried tomato. This dish will pair nicely with any variety, just make sure that the one you choose doesn't have any added sugar or other artificial ingredients.

INGREDIENTS | SERVES 6

6 cups water

1 (16-ounce) package brown rice pasta (any variety)

1 (12-ounce) package chicken sausage (no sugar added), sliced into ¼"-thick coins

2 cups chopped spinach

½ cup chopped roasted red peppers

Take It from Popeye

Spinach contains a unique antioxidant called lipoic acid that aids in the regeneration of vitamin C and vitamin E and can help regulate blood sugar levels.

1. Bring water to a boil in a large stockpot over medium-high heat. Cook pasta in boiling water 6–8 minutes or until pasta reaches desired consistency. Drain and set aside.

2. Heat a medium skillet over medium heat. Cook sausage in skillet until it browns. Add spinach and peppers to pan. Continue cooking until spinach wilts, about 3 minutes.

3. Pour sausage mixture over pasta.

Vegetable Rice Soup

Parsnips aren't as popular as they once were, but you should still be able to find them in most grocery stores. Choose parsnips that are white—the whiter the flesh, the sweeter the parsnip—and firm with intact roots. Avoid parsnips that are yellowing, browning, or look shriveled.

INGREDIENTS | SERVES 4

2 tablespoons water

1 medium yellow onion, peeled and chopped

2 cloves garlic, minced

2 stalks celery, chopped

2 medium carrots, peeled and chopped

1 cup sliced mushrooms

1 cup cubed parsnips

1 medium vine-ripened tomato, seeded and diced

6 cups vegetable broth

½ teaspoon dried parsley

¼ teaspoon dried thyme

½ teaspoon salt

½ teaspoon ground black pepper

¼ cup uncooked brown rice

1. In a large stockpot, heat water over medium heat. Add onion, garlic, celery, and carrots and cook until soft, about 5–6 minutes.

2. Add remaining ingredients except rice and bring to a boil over high heat. Boil 5 minutes and then reduce heat to medium-low.

3. Add uncooked rice and allow soup to simmer 45–60 minutes. Serve warm.

Potatoes versus Parsnips

Parsnips are similar to potatoes in texture and taste, but they have fewer natural sugars and more fiber. They're also richer in calcium.

Tomato Basil Chicken Linguini

Brown rice pasta is a popular choice with the gluten-free crowd because, unlike other wheat pasta alternatives, it has a mild flavor and can withstand longer cooking times.

INGREDIENTS | SERVES 4

6 cups plus 2 tablespoons water

8 ounces brown rice linguini

½ cup minced white onion

2 cloves garlic, minced

2 cups chopped fresh tomatoes

¼ cup chopped fresh basil

½ teaspoon salt

¼ teaspoon ground black pepper

½ teaspoon hot sauce

4 (4-ounce) boneless skinless chicken breasts, cubed

1. Bring 6 cups water to a boil in a large pot over medium-high heat and add brown rice linguini. Cook until pasta reaches desired consistency, about 6–8 minutes. Drain and set aside.

2. Heat 2 tablespoons water in a medium skillet over medium-high heat. Add onion and garlic and cook until translucent, about 5 minutes. Stir in tomatoes and cook 3 more minutes.

3. Add remaining ingredients and cook until chicken is no longer pink, about 8 minutes.

4. Pour chicken mixture over pasta and toss to combine. Serve immediately.

Spicy Garlic Chicken

This recipe pairs well with brown rice and roasted vegetables. Chop the chicken into cubes after cooking and toss with rice and broccoli to make it a spicy garlic rice bowl.

INGREDIENTS | SERVES 4

½ teaspoon salt
¼ teaspoon ground black pepper
¼ teaspoon onion powder
¼ teaspoon garlic powder
¼ teaspoon smoked paprika
⅛ teaspoon cayenne pepper
½ teaspoon dried parsley
4 (4-ounce) boneless skinless chicken breasts
½ fresh medium lime

1. Preheat oven to 350°F.

2. Combine salt, pepper, onion powder, garlic powder, paprika, cayenne, and parsley in a plastic gallon-sized bag. Shake to mix.

3. Put chicken in bag and shake bag to coat chicken.

4. Put chicken in a baking dish and bake 30 minutes or until chicken is cooked through and juices run clear. Remove from oven and squeeze lime over chicken breasts before serving.

CHAPTER 5

MD Stage 1 Snacks and Sides

Smashed Sweet Potatoes

Make sure to wash and scrub your potatoes before smashing and cooking,
since you'll be eating the delicious skin in this recipe.

INGREDIENTS | SERVES 4

2 large sweet potatoes, cut in half lengthwise
½ teaspoon salt
½ teaspoon ground cinnamon
¼ teaspoon ground nutmeg

Naturally Sweet

Don't let the sweetness in sweet potatoes fool you. Although they are sweet tasting, their natural sugars are slowly released into the bloodstream, which balances blood sugar and gives you a lasting source of energy without blood sugar spikes that are linked to "crashes" and weight gain.

1. Preheat oven to 400°F. Place sweet potatoes cut-side down on a baking sheet.

2. Bake 25 minutes or until potatoes are soft.

3. Remove potatoes from oven and transfer them to a medium bowl.

4. Smash sweet potatoes in their skin with a potato masher. Sprinkle salt, cinnamon, and nutmeg on top and smash again. Serve warm.

Roasted Beets

Select beets that feel heavy for their size and have no cuts in their flesh. If beets are
available with the greens still attached, you can use them as an indicator of freshness.
Wilted beet greens indicate that the beet is not as fresh as you'd want.

INGREDIENTS | SERVES 4

4 large beets, peeled and cut into cubes
1 teaspoon dried rosemary
¼ teaspoon sea salt

B is for Betalains

Beets are rich in unique phytonutrients called betalains, which have been shown to provide antioxidant, anti-inflammatory, and detoxification effects. Betalains may also lessen the growth of tumor cells.

1. Preheat oven to 425°F. Line a baking sheet with parchment paper.

2. Arrange beets in a single layer on baking sheet and sprinkle with rosemary and sea salt.

3. Roast 15 minutes or until beets are tender.

Quinoa Tabbouleh

Traditionally, tabbouleh is made of cracked wheat, tomatoes, onions, parsley, and olive oil. This version gives you all the flavor without the wheat and gluten.

INGREDIENTS | SERVES 6

1 cup quinoa, rinsed and drained
1½ cups water
½ teaspoon salt
3 tablespoons lemon juice
1 tablespoon lime juice
1 clove garlic, minced
2 tablespoons minced red onion
½ teaspoon ground black pepper
2 medium Persian cucumbers, diced
1 pint cherry tomatoes, cut into fourths
½ cup chopped parsley

1. Combine quinoa, water, and salt in a medium saucepan over medium-high heat. Bring to a boil, then cover and reduce heat to low. Simmer until water is absorbed and quinoa is tender, about 10–15 minutes. Remove from heat and let stand covered 5 more minutes. Fluff with a fork.

2. Combine remaining ingredients in a large bowl and mix well. Pour in quinoa and mix to coat. Let chill at least 1 hour before serving.

Baked Grapefruit

Choose grapefruit that are slightly reddish in color and whose skin bounces back when you press on it lightly. This indicates that the grapefruit is ripe and will be much more flavorful.

INGREDIENTS | SERVES 2

1 large pink grapefruit, cut in half
½ teaspoon ground cinnamon
½ teaspoon ground ginger
1 teaspoon granulated stevia

1. Preheat oven to 375°F.

2. Place grapefruit cut-side up on baking sheet. Sprinkle each half with ¼ teaspoon cinnamon, ¼ teaspoon ginger, and ½ teaspoon stevia.

3. Bake 15 minutes. Serve warm.

The Mighty Grapefruit

Grapefruit has long been a diet staple because of its low calorie count, but did you know that grapefruit contains a compound—a flavonoid called naringin— that may help control your weight and blood sugar levels?

Red Beans and Rice

The combination of rice and beans is often called the perfect protein because rice contains the amino acids that beans are missing and vice versa.

INGREDIENTS | SERVES 4

2 tablespoons chicken broth

1 small onion, peeled and diced

2 stalks celery, diced

1 teaspoon salt

½ teaspoon ground black pepper

⅛ teaspoon cayenne pepper

2 tablespoons chopped fresh parsley

½ teaspoon dried thyme

1 (15.5-ounce) can red kidney beans, drained and rinsed

2 cups cooked brown rice

1. Heat broth in a medium skillet over medium heat. Add onion and celery and cook until softened, about 5 minutes.

2. Add spices and beans and allow to cook 5 minutes. Stir in rice.

3. Serve warm.

Balsamic-Glazed Carrots

Look for carrots that are firm with a smooth skin and bright orange in color. Choose a bunch that contains medium-sized carrots instead of larger ones. Less mature carrots tend to be sweeter and more tender than larger, older carrots.

INGREDIENTS | SERVES 4

3 cups carrots

2 tablespoons balsamic vinegar

½ teaspoon salt

¼ teaspoon ground black pepper

½ teaspoon dried parsley

1. Preheat oven to 400°F. Line a baking sheet with parchment paper.

2. Toss carrots, vinegar, salt, and pepper together in a large mixing bowl. Spread carrots on baking sheet in an even layer.

3. Bake 30–40 minutes until carrots reach desired consistency. Remove from oven and sprinkle with parsley.

Cuckoo for Carrots

Carrots are often shunned on a weight-loss program because of their carbohydrate content, but most of the carbohydrates come from fiber. A specific type of soluble fiber in carrots—called calcium pectate—not only fills you up but can also lower blood cholesterol levels.

"Creamed" Spinach

This spinach recipe has all the texture of creamed spinach without the extra calories from full-fat dairy products like cream or cheese.

INGREDIENTS | SERVES 6

2 pounds fresh spinach
½ cup chicken broth, divided
2 garlic cloves, minced
1 small yellow onion, peeled and diced
½ teaspoon salt
Juice from 1 large lemon

Spinach Trick

Spinach is known for being sandy before washing. The most efficient way to get all of this sand off is to put the spinach in a strainer and then submerge it in a bowl of cold water. Give it a quick swish, and then let it sit for a minute. Pull the strainer up out of the water and repeat once more. Most of the sand will sink to the bottom of the water then wash away.

1. Steam spinach in a double boiler until completely wilted, about 3 minutes. Allow to cool and then squeeze out excess moisture.

2. Add 1 tablespoon broth to a medium skillet over medium heat; cook the garlic and onion until soft, about 5 minutes.

3. Put cooked spinach, garlic, and onion in a food processor with remaining broth, salt, and lemon juice. Process until smooth.

Spicy Baked Tortilla Chips

Making your own tortilla chips is so simple—and so tasty—that you'll never want to buy them premade again. Serve them with homemade guacamole or fresh salsa.

INGREDIENTS | SERVES 6

1 (12-ounce) package brown rice tortillas
2 tablespoons fresh lime juice
1 teaspoon ground cumin
½ teaspoon chili powder

1. Preheat oven to 350°F.

2. Cut each tortilla into 8 triangles and spread out in a single layer on a baking sheet. Drizzle with lime juice and then sprinkle cumin and chili powder on top.

3. Bake 15 minutes or until chips are crispy.

Black Bean Dip

This Black Bean Dip makes the perfect pairing with the Spicy Baked Tortilla Chips (see recipe in this chapter). Kick it up a notch by adding some minced jalapeños.

INGREDIENTS | SERVES 4

1 (15.5-ounce) can black beans, drained and rinsed

½ cup chopped yellow onion

2 cloves garlic, minced

1 teaspoon ground cumin

½ teaspoon chili powder

½ teaspoon salt

2 teaspoons tomato paste

1 tablespoon fresh lime juice

1 tablespoon chopped green chilies

2 green onions, chopped

¼ cup chopped cilantro

1. Put beans, onion, garlic, cumin, chili powder, salt, tomato paste, and lime juice in a food processor and process until smooth.

2. Stir in green chilies and garnish with green onions and cilantro.

Butyric Acid in Beans

Black beans provide special support for your digestive tract—and your colon especially. The indigestible portion of black beans contains the ideal mix of substances to feed the bacteria in your colon so that they're able to produce butyric acid. This butyric acid provides fuel to the cells in the lining of the colon and keeps the digestive tract functioning optimally.

Simple Quinoa

Rinse the quinoa well before cooking. Rinsing removes quinoa's natural outer coating—called saponin—that can make the quinoa taste soapy and bitter.

INGREDIENTS | SERVES 4

1 cup quinoa, rinsed and drained
2 cups vegetable broth
½ teaspoon garlic salt
1 teaspoon fresh lemon juice

1. Combine quinoa and broth in a medium saucepan over high heat. Bring to a boil and then reduce heat to low and cover. Allow to simmer 20 minutes or until quinoa is tender and fluffy.

2. Fluff quinoa with a fork and stir in garlic salt and lemon juice. Serve warm.

Fruit Salad

This refreshing Fruit Salad is a breeze to throw together. It satisfies any sweet craving while also providing you with essential vitamins and minerals that sugar-laden desserts don't.

INGREDIENTS | SERVES 4

1 cup diced cantaloupe
1 cup diced honeydew
1 cup diced pineapple
1 cup halved strawberries, hulled
1 teaspoon ground cinnamon
½ teaspoon granulated stevia

Combine all ingredients in a large bowl and toss to coat. Chill covered a minimum 30 minutes before serving.

Want a Flat Belly? Eat Pineapple!

Pineapple contains an enzyme called bromelain, which aids in the proper digestion of protein. It also is highly anti-inflammatory, so it can reduce swelling and make your belly appear flatter.

Turnip Fries

Look for small- to medium-sized turnips. Larger turnips tend to have a coarse texture with a bitter, woody taste, while smaller turnips are sweeter and more tender.

INGREDIENTS | SERVES 2

4 small turnips, peeled and cut into 2" sticks
¼ teaspoon salt
¼ teaspoon ground black pepper
¼ teaspoon chili powder

The Cruciferous Turnip

Turnips are often grouped with root vegetables like potatoes, but they actually belong to the cruciferous family—along with broccoli, Brussels sprouts, and kale. Just one medium-sized turnip provides more than half of the amount of vitamin C you need for an entire day.

1. Preheat oven to 425°F.

2. Place turnip sticks on a foil-lined baking pan.

3. Sprinkle salt, pepper, and chili powder over turnips and toss.

4. Spread out in a single layer. Bake in the oven 15 minutes, flip fries over, and then bake another 15 minutes. Serve warm.

Pumpkin Pie Apple Slices

This snack flawlessly combines two fall favorites—pumpkin pie and apple crisp—without any of the added sugar.

INGREDIENTS | SERVES 2

2 teaspoons pumpkin pie spice

1 teaspoon granulated stevia

2 medium Granny Smith apples, cored, and cut into thin slices

2 tablespoons lemon juice

2 tablespoons water

1. Combine pumpkin pie spice and stevia in a gallon-sized plastic bag. Place apple slices and lemon juice in a medium bowl and soak for 30 minutes; then put apple slices in plastic bag with pumpkin pie spice and shake until apples are covered.

2. Put water in a medium saucepan over medium heat and add coated apples. Cook 10 minutes or until apples are warm and tender. Serve warm.

Roast Beef and Pickle Wraps

When choosing a roast beef, ask the person at the deli counter if you can read the ingredient lists. You want to choose a meat that doesn't contain any added sugar or artificial ingredients.

INGREDIENTS | SERVES 2

4 slices (4 ounces) nitrate-free roast beef, sliced thinly

4 medium dill pickle spears

1. Cut each roast beef slice and each pickle spear in half.

2. Roll each pickle spear in roast beef and secure with a toothpick. Serve immediately.

Summer Squash Bake

This bake is done when the squash is fork tender, but still slightly crisp. Keep an eye on it as it bakes because overcooking can cause the squash to become soggy.

INGREDIENTS | SERVES 4

2 medium zucchini, sliced into ¼" rounds

2 medium yellow summer squash, sliced into ¼" rounds

2 teaspoons Italian seasoning

2 cloves garlic, minced

½ teaspoon salt

½ teaspoon ground black pepper

1. Preheat oven to 375°F.

2. Toss sliced zucchini and squash with seasoning, garlic, salt, and pepper in a medium bowl.

3. Pour onto a baking dish and bake 10 minutes. Flip over and then cook another 5 minutes or until softened.

Summer Squash for Sight

Summer squash is rich in two antioxidants—lutein and zeaxanthin—that are especially helpful in protecting eye health. Lutein and zeaxanthin protect against both age-related macular degeneration and cataracts.

Mashed Parsnips

If you want to add a little variety and raise the nutrient content of this side dish, opt for two pounds of parsnips and two pounds of turnips and mix the two together.

INGREDIENTS | SERVES 6

4 pounds parsnips, peeled and quartered
1 cup chicken broth
1 teaspoon salt
½ teaspoon ground black pepper
2 tablespoons chives

1. Put parsnips in a large stockpot with just enough water to cover. Bring to a boil over high heat and then reduce heat to low and simmer until parsnips are soft, about 20 minutes. Drain.

2. Put parsnips in a food processor with broth, salt, and pepper and process until smooth.

3. Stir in chives. Serve immediately.

Garlic Zucchini Noodles

Zucchini noodles cook very quickly, so don't go far from the stove when making this dish. You can test the noodles as they cook, and remove them from the heat quickly when they reach your desired level of doneness.

INGREDIENTS | SERVES 4

6 medium zucchini, julienned or cut into spirals with a spiralizer
1 teaspoon salt
1 tablespoon chicken broth
2 cloves garlic, minced

1. Sprinkle zucchini with salt and let "sweat" 30 minutes. Drain zucchini on a paper towel.

2. Heat broth in a medium skillet over medium heat. Add garlic and cook until fragrant, about 3 minutes.

3. Add zucchini "noodles" and cook until tender, about 5 minutes. Be careful not to overcook.

Z for Zoodles

Zucchini noodles, often referred to as "zoodles," are a breeze to make. They're even easier with a specialized vegetable cutter known as a spiralizer. A spiralizer cuts the zucchini into noodle-like strands that look just like pasta.

Mexican Brown Rice

If you want a little less spice, you can replace the fire-roasted tomatoes in this recipe with regular diced tomatoes or chopped fresh tomatoes. If you want some more spice, add some pickled jalapeños.

INGREDIENTS | SERVES 4

1 cup brown rice
1½ cups water
½ teaspoon salt
½ (15.5-ounce) can fire-roasted diced tomatoes
¼ cup chopped cilantro

1. Combine rice, water, and salt in a medium saucepan. Bring to a boil over high heat then cover and reduce heat to low. Allow to simmer 20 minutes or until water is absorbed and rice is soft. Remove from heat and fluff with a fork.

2. Add tomatoes and cilantro and stir until combined.

Sausage and Apple Stuffing

You won't even miss the bread in this gluten-free stuffing recipe. The sage gives it a traditional flavor, while the sweet potatoes add some bulk.

INGREDIENTS | SERVES 4

2 small sweet potatoes, peeled and diced

2 medium Granny Smith apples, cored and diced

1 tablespoon water

1 small yellow onion, peeled and diced

2 celery stalks, diced

½ pound Italian sausage, casings removed

½ teaspoon salt

½ teaspoon ground black pepper

½ teaspoon ground sage

An Apple a Day

The nondigestible compounds in apples can help fight obesity—and the health problems related to it, like diabetes, heart disease, and stroke. Granny Smith apples promote the growth of the good bacteria in the colon by providing them with the food they need to survive and multiply.

1. Preheat oven to 400°F. Line a baking sheet with parchment paper.

2. Toss diced sweet potatoes and apples together and spread in a single layer on the baking sheet. Roast until tender and slightly browned, about 30 minutes.

3. Heat water in a medium skillet over medium-high heat. Add onion and celery and cook until softened, about 5 minutes.

4. Add sausage, salt, pepper, and sage and cook until sausage is no longer pink, about 7 minutes.

5. Allow sausage to cool 5 minutes and then combine with sweet potato and apple mixture and toss to mix.

Quinoa Pilaf

This Quinoa Pilaf gives the traditional rice pilaf a run for its money.
It's a great side dish for any grainless entrée.

INGREDIENTS | SERVES 2

3 cups plus 2 tablespoons chicken broth
1 small shallot, peeled and minced
½ cup sliced white mushrooms
2 medium carrots, peeled and chopped
1½ cups quinoa, rinsed and drained
1 teaspoon salt
½ teaspoon ground black pepper
¼ cup chopped fresh parsley

1. Heat 2 tablespoons broth in a medium saucepan over medium heat. Add shallots and cook until softened, about 3 minutes. Add mushrooms and carrots and continue to cook until softened, about 5 minutes.

2. Add remaining broth and quinoa and stir until combined. Bring to a boil over high heat and then reduce heat to low and cover. Allow to simmer 20 minutes or until quinoa is tender and fluffy.

3. Fluff with a fork and then stir in salt, pepper, and parsley. Serve warm.

CHAPTER 6

MD Stage 1 Dessert

Berry Salad with Cacao Nibs

Cacao nibs not only add some crunch while giving this berry salad a rich, chocolate flavor, but they're also a rich source of vitamins, minerals, antioxidants, and fiber.

INGREDIENTS | SERVES 4

½ cup water

½ teaspoon granulated stevia

Juice from 1 medium lemon

1 teaspoon lemon zest

½ teaspoon vanilla extract

1 cup sliced strawberries

1 cup blueberries

1 cup raspberries

¼ cup cacao nibs

2 tablespoons chopped fresh mint leaves

1. Put water, stevia, lemon juice, vanilla extract, and lemon zest in a small saucepan. Stir and bring to a boil over high heat. Allow to boil 1 minute then turn heat to low and simmer 20 minutes. Remove from heat and transfer to the refrigerator. Refrigerate until cool.

2. Mix berries and cacao nibs together in a large bowl. Pour chilled syrup over fruit mixture and toss to coat. Sprinkle with mint leaves and toss to combine.

Tropical Cacao

Cacao nibs are known as "nature's chocolate chips" because they come from the pure cacao beans that come directly out of the cacao fruit. Cacao nibs are a better choice than chocolate chips because they don't have any of the added sugar or soy that most commercial chocolate chips do.

Strawberry Mug Cake

Mug cakes make the ideal dessert because they're ready in minutes, there're no leftovers to tempt you, and cleanup is a cinch!

INGREDIENTS | SERVES 1

2 tablespoons almond flour

½ tablespoon coconut flour

1 tablespoon unsweetened rice milk

1 large egg white

2 tablespoons mashed strawberries

¼ teaspoon baking powder

¼ teaspoon vanilla extract

⅛ teaspoon salt

Go Organic

Strawberries top the list of the dirtiest conventional produce because of their high exposure to pesticides. If you have to choose one thing to buy organic, make it strawberries.

1. Combine all ingredients in a mug and whisk with a fork to combine.

2. Microwave 90 seconds or until cake is set and a toothpick inserted in the center comes out clean.

Blueberry-Poached Apples

*Poaching these apples in a fresh blueberry mixture instead of
plain water gives them a flavor that can't be beat.*

INGREDIENTS | SERVES 4

2 cups frozen blueberries
1½ cups water
½ cup coconut water
1 teaspoon granulated stevia
4 medium Gala apples, peeled
and cored

1. Combine blueberries, water, coconut water, and stevia in a blender and blend until smooth. Strain through a cheesecloth and pour into a large pot.

2. Place apples in the blueberry mixture. Turn heat to medium-low and allow the liquid to come to a simmer. Simmer apples 20–25 minutes or until they're soft but not mushy.

3. Remove apples from mixture, reserving blueberry liquid in pot.

4. Turn heat to medium and allow liquid to reduce until it thickens a bit. Pour mixture over poached apples. Serve immediately.

Ginger Mango Sorbet

When selecting fresh ginger at the store, look for one that has firm, heavy "hands"—the pieces that are sticking off the thicker root. Avoid gingerroot that looks wrinkled or moldy.

INGREDIENTS | SERVES 4

1½ cups water

1 (1") piece fresh ginger, peeled

1 teaspoon lemon zest

1¾ cups coconut water

¼ cup freshly squeezed orange juice

1 cup mango purée

3 tablespoons lemon juice

Sans Ice Cream Maker

If you don't have an ice cream maker, you can still make this sweet treat and all other sorbets and ice cream by following these steps: Spread mixture in a freezer-safe dish and put in the freezer for a half-hour. Remove from freezer and stir and then return to freezer. Repeat these steps every 30–60 minutes until sorbet/ice cream reaches desired consistency.

1. Combine water, ginger, lemon zest, and coconut water in a medium saucepan. Bring mixture to a boil over high heat and then reduce heat to low and allow to simmer 20 minutes. Strain through a cheesecloth to remove zest and ginger piece.

2. Transfer liquid to blender and add orange juice, mango purée, and lemon juice. Blend until smooth. Transfer to a baking dish and allow to cool in the refrigerator at least 2 hours.

3. Transfer mixture to ice cream maker and freeze according to manufacturer's instructions.

Pineapple Coconut Popsicles

Fruit popsicles are an ideal treat for hot summer days. They're cooling, easy to make, and full of vitamins and minerals. Plus, the possibilities of combinations are endless.

INGREDIENTS | SERVES 4

1 cup diced pineapple
¾ cup coconut water
3 or 4 drops liquid stevia

1. Combine all ingredients in a blender. Blend until smooth.

2. Pour into popsicle molds and freeze.

Sans Popsicle Mold

If you don't have a popsicle mold, you can make these popsicles—and any other popsicles—by pouring the mixture into small paper cups and sticking a wooden craft stick in the center. Freeze until solid and then peel the paper cup away from the popsicle.

Green Pops

Making these pops in two steps gives them an appealing look when they're finished, but you could blend all the ingredients together and freeze like that, if desired.

INGREDIENTS | SERVES 2

2 medium kiwifruit, peeled
½ cup cubed frozen mango
½ cup sliced frozen peaches
1 cup coconut water
½ cup baby spinach

1. Blend kiwi in a blender or food processor. Pour evenly into the bottom of each open cavity in a popsicle mold.

2. Blend remaining ingredients together until smooth. Pour on top of kiwi.

3. Freeze.

Pumpkin Pie Smoothie

If you don't have pumpkin pie spice on hand, you can achieve the same flavor profile by combining cinnamon, ginger, cloves, nutmeg, and allspice.

INGREDIENTS | SERVES 2

¾ cup pumpkin purée

1 cup coconut water

1 teaspoon pumpkin pie spice

¼ teaspoon vanilla extract

¼ cup ice cubes

3 or 4 drops liquid stevia

⅛ teaspoon ground cinnamon

1. Put all ingredients except cinnamon in a blender and blend until smooth.

2. Sprinkle cinnamon on top.

Pick the Pure

All vanilla extract is not created equal. Pure vanilla extract is made by soaking vanilla bean pods in alcohol to extract their natural flavor. Imitation vanilla extract is created from vanillin, which is generally artificially made. Go for the real vanilla extract whenever possible.

Lemon Mug Cake

Don't skip the lemon zest in this recipe. Just a little bit of zest really amps up the lemon flavor in this cake.

INGREDIENTS | SERVES 1

2 large egg whites
2 tablespoons unsweetened rice milk
2 tablespoons fresh lemon juice
1 teaspoon grated lemon zest
½ teaspoon liquid stevia
2 tablespoons coconut flour
¼ teaspoon baking powder
⅛ teaspoon salt

1. Combine egg whites, rice milk, lemon juice, lemon zest, and stevia together in a mug. Whisk to combine.

2. In a separate small bowl, combine coconut flour, baking powder, and salt.

3. Add dry ingredients to wet ingredients in mug and mix well.

4. Microwave 90 seconds or until cake is set and toothpick inserted in center comes out clean.

Make Your Own!

Many commercially made rice milks contain added sugars and artificial ingredients. You can easily make your own at home by blending 1 cup of cooked brown rice with 4 cups of filtered water. Once the mixture is smooth, strain it with a nut bag and you're done!

Baked Cinnamon Apples

A little stevia goes a long way. One-half teaspoon of granulated stevia is equivalent in sweetness to about two teaspoons of sugar.

INGREDIENTS | SERVES 4

4 medium Granny Smith apples, peeled, cored, and sliced into thin slices

1 tablespoon ground cinnamon

1 teaspoon ground nutmeg

½ teaspoon granulated stevia

½ cup water

1. Preheat oven to 350°F.

2. Line the bottom of a 9" × 9" baking dish with the apple slices. Sprinkle with cinnamon, nutmeg, and stevia.

3. Pour water over apples and bake uncovered 30 minutes or until apples are tender but not mushy. Serve immediately.

Nature's Sweetener

Stevia is a green, leafy plant that has been used for centuries for its medicinal properties. It's more than just a no-calorie sweetener; stevia may also help lower blood sugar levels, fight diabetes, and reduce high blood pressure.

Blueberry Ginger Smoothie

This smoothie is sweet enough to be a dessert, but it's also energizing enough to be a quick, light breakfast.

INGREDIENTS | SERVES 2

1 cup blueberries
Juice from 1 medium lemon
1 (1") piece ginger, peeled
1 cup coconut water
1 teaspoon spirulina

Put all ingredients in a blender and blend until smooth. Serve immediately.

Spirulina the Superfood

Spirulina is a blue-green algae that's considered one of the oldest forms of life on Earth. It's often touted as one of the original superfoods. It's one of the only plant sources of complete protein and is rich in beta carotene, linoleic acid, arachidonic acid, iron, calcium, and vitamin B_{12}. It provides an almost instant increase in energy and may help increase endurance.

Lemon-Infused Strawberries

You can use this same infusion technique for any berries—blueberries, blackberries, and raspberries all make a great combination with the lemon.

INGREDIENTS | SERVES 4

1 pound fresh strawberries, hulled and halved
1 teaspoon granulated stevia
2 teaspoons lemon juice
1 teaspoon ground cinnamon, plus ¼ teaspoon for garnish

Combine strawberries, stevia, lemon juice, and 1 teaspoon cinnamon in a large bowl and stir. Let stand until strawberries start to break down, about 10 minutes. Sprinkle with remaining cinnamon.

Spiced Orange Slices

There are several types of oranges, and any will do well in this recipe, but if you're looking for a really juicy dessert, opt for Valencia oranges.

INGREDIENTS | SERVES 4

4 medium oranges, peeled, white pith removed, cut into thin slices

2 tablespoons freshly squeezed orange juice

2 tablespoons lemon juice

½ teaspoon granulated stevia

½ teaspoon ground cinnamon

⅛ teaspoon ground cloves

1. Arrange orange slices in a serving dish in a single layer.

2. In a small bowl, whisk together orange juice, lemon juice, stevia, cinnamon, and cloves.

3. Pour mixture over orange slices. Let sit 10 minutes before serving.

Orange You Glad

Oranges are most well known for their high vitamin C content—one medium Valencia orange contains 97 percent of the amount of vitamin C you need for the whole day. Vitamin C is a powerful antioxidant that neutralizes free radicals and helps protect cells from damage that can cause cancer and heart disease.

Blackberry Lemon Sorbet

*Allowing the frozen blackberries to slightly defrost—but not thaw completely—
before making this sorbet will give you a smooth consistency that's not too icy.*

INGREDIENTS | SERVES 4

2 cups frozen blackberries
Juice from 1 medium lemon
Zest from 1 medium lemon
⅓ cup water
7–10 drops liquid stevia

1. Allow blackberries to defrost slightly. Combine all ingredients in a blender and blend until smooth.

2. Pour mixture into an ice cream maker and freeze according to manufacturer's instructions.

3. Serve immediately.

Mango Smoothie

*You can use fresh mango in this recipe in place of frozen. If you do, add a few
ice cubes to thicken the smoothie and get the proper texture.*

INGREDIENTS | SERVES 2

1 cup frozen mango cubes
¼ cup coconut water
¾ cup unsweetened rice milk
1 medium orange, peeled and sliced

Combine all ingredients in a blender. Blend until smooth.

The Mighty Mango

Mangoes contain tartaric acid, malic acid, and a small amount of citric acid—which all help alkalize the body. An alkalized body contributes to better digestion, increased mental alertness, more energy, and better sleep.

Strawberry Kiwi Pops

Choose your kiwifruit by holding it between your thumb and forefinger and applying gentle pressure. You want a kiwifruit that gives a little but is not mushy. Avoid any that have bruised or soft spots or shriveled skin.

INGREDIENTS | SERVES 4

⅔ cup chopped kiwifruit

⅔ cup chopped strawberries

½ cup coconut water

1. Combine kiwi and strawberries in a medium bowl. Divide fruit mixture evenly between four popsicle molds.

2. Pour coconut water on top of fruit. Freeze.

The Small, Green Vitamin C Machine

Oranges are often thought of as the vitamin C powerhouse, but kiwifruit gives them a run for their money. One serving of kiwifruit has two and a half times the amount of vitamin C you need for the entire day.

Spiced Pear Sorbet

Each variety of pear has its own distinct flavor and texture. Anjou pears are mellow in flavor, yet big in juiciness. If you can't find Anjou pears for this recipe, choose Bartlett, which is mild with subtle citrus notes.

INGREDIENTS | SERVES 4

1 pound Anjou pears, peeled and cored

¾ cup coconut water

⅔ cup water

1–2 teaspoons granulated stevia

1 teaspoon Chinese five-spice powder

1 whole star anise

1 small cinnamon stick

2 orange slices

1 teaspoon orange zest

1. Combine all ingredients in a large saucepan and cook over medium-high heat about 30 minutes or until pears start to turn mushy.

2. Remove cinnamon stick and orange slices and process ingredients in a food processor until smooth.

3. Pour into a baking dish and refrigerate until cool, at least 1 hour to overnight.

4. Once mixture has cooled, pour into ice cream maker and freeze according to manufacturer's instructions. Serve immediately.

Chocolate Coffee Smoothie

You can use coffee-flavored extract or an all-natural coffee-flavored liquid stevia in place of the instant coffee granules in this recipe without compromising any flavor.

INGREDIENTS | SERVES 2

1 cup unsweetened rice milk

1 tablespoon unsweetened cocoa powder

1 teaspoon vanilla extract

2 cups ice

2 teaspoons instant coffee granules

2 or 3 drops liquid stevia

Combine all ingredients in a blender and blend until smooth.

Fruit Kebabs

Allowing these fruit kebabs to sit for a couple minutes with the granulated stevia on top will pull some of the fruit's water out and give the fruit a really juicy flavor.

INGREDIENTS | SERVES 4

10 large strawberries, halved and hulled

1 cup cubed pineapple

1 cup cubed cantaloupe

1 cup cubed honeydew melon

2 kiwifruit, peeled and sliced

1 teaspoon granulated stevia

Thread fruit onto skewers. Arrange on a serving plate and sprinkle with stevia. Let sit 2 minutes before serving.

Blueberry Lime Sorbet

With just four simple ingredients, you can have a fresh sorbet whipped up in less than an hour.

INGREDIENTS | SERVES 4

4 cups blueberries
1 medium lime, juiced and zested
½ teaspoon liquid stevia
1 cup coconut water

Hydrate with Coconut Water

Coconut water is one of nature's best hydrators. It's rich in potassium and low in sodium, unlike commercially produced sports drinks that are made for the same purpose.

1. Place all ingredients in a blender and blend until smooth.

2. Pour mixture into an ice cream maker and freeze according to manufacturer's instructions.

3. Serve immediately.

Chocolate Mug Cake

You won't even be able to taste the pumpkin in this recipe. It's just there to give a smooth, cake-like consistency to this quick, simple mug cake.

INGREDIENTS | SERVES 1

2 large egg whites
¼ cup pumpkin purée
2 tablespoons almond flour
1 tablespoon granulated stevia
1 tablespoon unsweetened cocoa powder
¼ teaspoon baking powder
¼ teaspoon vanilla extract
⅛ teaspoon salt
1 teaspoon unsweetened rice milk

1. Combine all ingredients in a mug, making sure to mix thoroughly so there are no chunks or powder left over.

2. Microwave 2 minutes or until cake is set.

3. Serve immediately.

MD Stage 2 Breakfast

Egg White Scramble

This breakfast is so easy you can whip it up on any busy day. Make it your own by adding any nonstarchy vegetables, like broccoli, asparagus, or kale.

INGREDIENTS | SERVES 2

2 teaspoons olive oil

2 tablespoons minced yellow onion

2 tablespoons minced garlic

2 tablespoons minced green bell pepper

½ cup chopped white mushrooms

1 cup chopped spinach

6 large egg whites

1 teaspoon salt

1 teaspoon ground black pepper

½ teaspoon red pepper flakes (optional)

1. Heat olive oil in a medium skillet over medium heat and add onion, garlic, and green pepper.

2. Sauté until soft, about 5 minutes. Add mushrooms and cook another 5 minutes or until mushrooms soften.

3. Stir in spinach and cook until wilted, about 3 minutes. Add egg whites, salt, pepper, and red pepper if desired and scramble until eggs reach desired consistency. Serve warm.

Denver Omelet

Denver—or western—omelets are a staple on most breakfast menus. With this recipe, you can make your own healthy version at home.

INGREDIENTS | SERVES 2

1 teaspoon olive oil

½ cup minced red onion

¼ cup chopped green bell pepper

¼ cup chopped red bell pepper

2 slices deli ham (no sugar added), chopped

4 large eggs, whisked

¼ teaspoon salt

¼ teaspoon ground black pepper

Watch Your Ham

Many deli hams have brown sugar added to give it that "honey ham" flavor. Look for a cubed ham that doesn't have sugar or any other artificial ingredients.

1. Heat olive oil in a medium skillet over low heat.

2. When oil is hot, add onion and peppers and sauté until vegetables are soft, about 4 minutes.

3. Add ham to mixture and cook until heated through, about 2 minutes.

4. In a small bowl, whisk eggs together with salt and pepper.

5. Add whisked eggs on top of mixture and allow to cook on one side. Once eggs are cooked on bottom, about 4 minutes, flip over and allow to cook on the other side, about 3 minutes. Once eggs are cooked, flip in half to make an omelet. Serve warm.

Bacon and Egg "Muffins"

You can make these "muffins" up to a week in advance and store them in a bag in the refrigerator. They make a great grab-and-go breakfast for the workweek.

INGREDIENTS | SERVES 6

12 large eggs
1 cup finely chopped cooked broccoli
6 slices cooked turkey bacon, chopped
½ teaspoon salt
¼ teaspoon ground black pepper

1. Preheat oven to 350°F. Line twelve-cup muffin pan with cupcake liners.

2. Whisk all ingredients together in a large bowl. Pour mixture evenly between each well of the muffin pan.

3. Bake 20–25 minutes or until egg is set. Remove egg cups from pan and allow to cool on a baking rack.

Chicken Sausage with Spinach and Zucchini

This recipe challenges the traditional breakfast by not including any eggs or other foods typically associated with breakfast. Go out of your breakfast comfort zone by trying foods that you wouldn't normally eat for breakfast at least twice a week.

INGREDIENTS | SERVES 2

2 teaspoons olive oil
2 chicken sausage links, roughly chopped
1 large zucchini, diced
2 cups chopped spinach
½ teaspoon salt
¼ teaspoon ground black pepper

1. Heat olive oil in a medium skillet over medium-high heat and add sausage. Sauté until browned and crisp, about 8 minutes.

2. Add zucchini and cook until softened, about 4 minutes. Add spinach and cook until wilted, about 3 minutes. Sprinkle on salt and pepper and stir until combined.

3. Serve immediately.

Spicy Scrambled Eggs

Eating spicy eggs in the morning gets your metabolism going straight out of the gate. If you're not into spice, omit the jalapeño and dial back on the hot sauce.

INGREDIENTS | SERVES 2

2 teaspoons olive oil

½ small jalapeño pepper, seeded and finely minced

½ cup chopped red pepper

2 large eggs

3 large egg whites

⅛ teaspoon ground cumin

¼ teaspoon salt

¼ teaspoon ground black pepper

1 teaspoon hot sauce

Make It Spicy!

Hot sauce has been shown to increase metabolism for hours after you eat a meal. The capsaicin in hot sauce—the compound responsible for this effect—also works as a blood thinner, helping to prevent blood clots.

1. Heat olive oil in a medium skillet over medium-high heat. Add both peppers and sauté until softened, about 5–6 minutes.

2. In a medium bowl, beat together eggs, egg whites, cumin, salt, and black pepper. Pour eggs over peppers and scramble until eggs are cooked, another 3–4 minutes. Top with hot sauce.

Turkey Bacon and Egg Wrap

Turkey bacon is a lower-fat alternative to the traditional, greasy pork bacon. Choose one that is nitrate-free and doesn't contain any fillers.

INGREDIENTS | SERVES 2

2 teaspoons avocado oil

4 slices turkey bacon, chopped

4 large eggs

½ teaspoon salt

¼ teaspoon ground black pepper

¼ cup chopped roasted red peppers

2 large iceberg lettuce leaves

½ medium avocado, pitted, flesh removed, and sliced thinly

A+ for Avocado Oil

Avocado oil is ideal for high-heat cooking because it stands up to higher temperatures than some other popular oils, like olive. Avocado oil is made up of 50 percent monounsaturated fats.

1. Heat avocado oil in a medium skillet over medium-high heat and add bacon.

2. While bacon is cooking, beat together eggs, salt, and black pepper in a small bowl. When bacon is cooked, add eggs and scramble until almost cooked. Add red pepper and continue cooking until eggs are cooked through.

3. Lay lettuce leaves flat and fill each with half the egg mixture. Top with half the avocado and roll up like a wrap. Secure with a toothpick and serve immediately.

Breakfast Sausage and Peppers

Sausage and peppers are popular for lunch and dinner, but when you try this recipe, you'll be hooked on it for breakfast too.

INGREDIENTS | SERVES 2

1 tablespoon olive oil

1 large green bell pepper, seeded and cut into strips

1 large red bell pepper, seeded and cut into strips

1 small yellow onion, peeled and sliced

1 pound ground pork

1 teaspoon salt

¼ teaspoon garlic salt

½ teaspoon dried parsley

¼ teaspoon dried thyme

¼ teaspoon red pepper flakes

¾ teaspoon ground sage

¼ teaspoon coarsely ground black pepper

¼ teaspoon ground coriander

⅛ teaspoon dried oregano

1. Heat olive oil in a large skillet over medium-high heat and add peppers and onion. Sauté until softened, about 5–7 minutes.

2. Add ground pork and seasonings and cook until pork is no longer pink.

3. Serve immediately.

Chemoprotective Parsley

Parsley is often written off as a garnish, but the green is extremely powerful. Parsley contains a compound called myricetin, which has been shown to help prevent the development of skin cancer.

Eggs with Smoked Salmon

*Pairing some smoked salmon with your morning eggs is a good way to get
a head start on your intake of omega-3 fatty acids for the day.*

INGREDIENTS | SERVES 2

1 teaspoon avocado oil

⅓ cup chopped yellow onion

½ cup halved cherry tomatoes

4 ounces smoked salmon

4 large eggs

¼ teaspoon ground black pepper

¼ teaspoon celery salt

1 tablespoon chopped fresh parsley

1. Heat avocado oil in a medium skillet over medium heat. Add onion and sauté until translucent, about 4 minutes.

2. Add cherry tomatoes and smoked salmon and cook until heated through, about 3 minutes.

3. Add eggs, pepper, and celery salt and scramble until cooked through, about 4 minutes.

4. Remove from heat and top with parsley. Serve immediately.

Nutty N'oatmeal

Just because you can't have oats in Stage 2 of this program doesn't mean you can't enjoy a warm, porridge-like breakfast. This "oatmeal" is made with different types of nuts and flaxseed that are cooked down to give it a creamy texture.

INGREDIENTS | SERVES 2

¼ cup crushed raw walnut pieces

¼ cup crushed raw almond pieces

2 tablespoons ground flaxseed

1 cup unsweetened almond milk

2 teaspoons chia seeds

½ teaspoon ground cinnamon

¼ teaspoon ground nutmeg

1 teaspoon granulated stevia

1. Add walnut, almond, and flaxseed to a small saucepan and stir over medium heat until toasted, about 5 minutes.

2. Add milk, chia seeds, cinnamon, and nutmeg and allow to cook 7 minutes, stirring occasionally. Remove from heat and stir in stevia. Serve immediately.

The Mighty Flax

Flaxseed offers a wide range of health benefits, but its three most notable are its high content of omega-3 fatty acids, fiber, and lignans. Lignans help reduce the rate of reproductive and colon cancer, improve heart health, and increase hair growth.

Frittata with Mixed Greens

Using a variety of mixed greens in this recipe optimizes nutrient intake,
but you can use whatever greens you have on hand.

INGREDIENTS | SERVES 4

3 tablespoons olive oil

2 cloves garlic, minced

1 medium yellow onion, peeled
and chopped

6 cups mixed greens (kale, Swiss chard,
spinach, collard greens), chopped into
bite-sized pieces

8 large eggs

½ teaspoon salt

½ teaspoon ground black pepper

½ cup chopped fresh basil leaves

¼ teaspoon red pepper flakes

2 teaspoons hot sauce

1. Preheat oven to 350°F.

2. Heat olive oil in a medium skillet over medium-high heat. Add garlic and onion and sauté until translucent, about 3–4 minutes. Add greens to skillet and cook until wilted, about 5 minutes.

3. In a medium bowl, beat together eggs with salt, pepper, basil, and red pepper flakes. Fold in wilted greens.

4. Pour egg mixture into a 9" × 9" baking dish. Bake 25–30 minutes or until eggs are set.

5. Remove from oven and dash with hot sauce before serving.

Expand Your Greens

Swiss chard—also called Roman kale, silverbeet, and strawberry spinach—is an excellent source of vitamins A, K, and C. It's also rich in lutein and zeaxanthin, which protect your retinas from any age-related damage.

Sausage Breakfast Muffins

These Sausage Breakfast Muffins can be made up to a week in advance and stored in the refrigerator. If you want to make them even further in advance, freeze them after cooking and thaw as needed.

INGREDIENTS | SERVES 2

½ pound ground pork sausage
12 large eggs
1 small white onion, peeled and finely diced
1 teaspoon garlic powder
½ teaspoon salt
¼ teaspoon ground black pepper
1 tablespoon Italian seasoning
½ cup sliced mushrooms
2 green onions, chopped

1. Preheat oven to 350°F. Line a twelve-cup muffin tray with cupcake liners.

2. Put sausage in a medium skillet and cook over medium heat until no longer pink, about 7 minutes. Drain.

3. In a large bowl, combine remaining ingredients and beat until combined. Add sausage and stir.

4. Scoop ¼ cup egg mixture into each muffin cup and bake 20 minutes or until egg has set.

Avocado Boats

Take these stuffed avocados out of the oven as soon as the egg is cooked through. If you cook an avocado too long, it develops a bitter, unpleasant taste.

INGREDIENTS | SERVES 2

2 large avocados, halved lengthwise and pitted

4 strips cooked turkey bacon, crumbled

4 large eggs

¼ teaspoon sea salt

¼ teaspoon ground black pepper

Your Fatty Friend

Avocados are marveled for their high content of healthy fats. It's not just the fat itself that's beneficial; it's what the fat does for you. The monounsaturated fat in avocados helps you absorb carotenoids—plant pigments with incredible health benefits—more effectively.

1. Preheat oven to 400°F.

2. Scoop some avocado out of each half to create a well.

3. Sprinkle bacon equally into each avocado well. Crack 1 egg directly into each avocado half. Season with salt and pepper.

4. Bake 15 minutes on a baking sheet or until egg is cooked to desired doneness.

Cinnamon "Oatmeal"

This is another version of "oatmeal" that contains absolutely no oats; however, instead of nuts, this recipe uses chia seeds and ground flaxseed.

INGREDIENTS | SERVES 1

½ cup unsweetened coconut milk

¼ cup chia seeds

¼ cup ground flaxseed

3 tablespoons unsweetened shredded coconut

1 teaspoon ground cinnamon

1 teaspoon granulated stevia

1. Heat coconut milk in a small saucepan over medium heat. Add remaining ingredients and stir until incorporated.

2. Remove from heat and allow mixture to sit 5 minutes or until liquid is absorbed.

Grind As Needed

Because ground flaxseed is so high in fat content, it goes rancid fairly easily. It's best to purchase whole flaxseed and then grind it with a coffee grinder as needed. The shell of the whole flaxseed protects it from going rancid.

Packed Vegetable Omelet

This recipe is for your basic vegetable omelet, but you can adjust it to your own taste by swapping out any of the vegetables for your favorite Stage 2–approved ones.

INGREDIENTS | SERVES 2

1 tablespoon plus 1 teaspoon olive oil

½ cup sliced mushrooms

10 cherry tomatoes, halved

½ cup spinach

½ cup cooked chopped broccoli

4 large eggs

½ teaspoon salt

¼ teaspoon ground black pepper

¼ teaspoon garlic powder

¼ teaspoon red pepper flakes

Fresh versus Frozen

Keeping fresh vegetables on hand at all times can be difficult. Stock your freezer with frozen vegetables and use them in recipes like this one. Frozen vegetables are often less expensive than fresh ones and may be even more nutritious. Some vitamins are lost directly after picking the vegetable. Freezing immediately after picking stops this vitamin loss.

1. Heat 1 tablespoon olive oil in an 8" skillet over medium-high heat. Add mushrooms and sauté until softened, about 4 minutes. Add tomatoes and spinach and continue cooking until spinach wilts, about 3 minutes. Add broccoli and cook until heated through, about 4 minutes. Remove vegetables from pan and set aside.

2. Heat remaining 1 teaspoon olive oil in the same skillet over medium heat. In a small bowl, beat eggs with salt, pepper, garlic powder, and red pepper flakes. Add eggs to hot pan and allow to cook until eggs start to set, about 6 minutes.

3. Flip eggs over and cook the other side. While eggs are cooking, scoop vegetables onto half the cooked egg. Flip the other half over to form an omelet.

4. Remove from heat, cut in half, and serve immediately.

Breakfast Stuffed Peppers

Make sure to add the egg to these stuffed peppers only after they have already baked for a while. If you add them too early, the eggs will get overdone before the peppers are even softened.

INGREDIENTS | SERVES 2

2 medium bell peppers, halved and seeded

2 tablespoons olive oil

½ cup sliced mushrooms

¼ cup chopped yellow onion

1½ cups baby spinach

½ teaspoon garlic salt

¼ teaspoon ground black pepper

4 large eggs

1. Preheat oven to 375°F. Line a baking sheet with parchment paper. Arrange peppers cut-side up on baking sheet.

2. Heat olive oil in a medium skillet over medium-high heat. Add mushrooms and onion and sauté until soft, about 5 minutes. Add spinach, garlic salt, and pepper and cook until wilted, about 3 minutes.

3. Scoop vegetable mixture into each pepper "cup." Bake 20 minutes.

4. Remove from oven and crack an egg on top of each pepper half. Return to oven and bake another 15 minutes or until egg has set. Serve immediately.

Breakfast Pizza

You won't really be eating pizza for breakfast, but the Italian herbs, tomatoes, and red pepper flakes will give you the flavor without the carbohydrate load.

INGREDIENTS | SERVES 2

1½ teaspoons olive oil

2 large eggs, lightly beaten

¼ teaspoon dried oregano

¼ teaspoon dried basil

⅛ teaspoon red pepper flakes

5 grape tomatoes

2 slices cooked turkey bacon, crumbled

1 tablespoon sliced black olives

1. Heat oil in an 8" skillet over medium heat. Add eggs and seasonings and allow to cook until eggs start to set, about 3 minutes.

2. Arrange remaining ingredients on top and allow egg to finish cooking. Fold in half and serve immediately.

Help Hair with Olives

Black olives are rich in vitamin E—one of the most powerful antioxidant vitamins. They also contain fatty acids that nourish, hydrate, and protect the hair and skin.

Grain-Free Granola

You can eat this Grain-Free Granola dry or put it in a bowl and top it with coconut milk, almond milk, or rice milk for a grain-free cereal that will keep you full until lunch.

INGREDIENTS | SERVES 8

1½ cups crushed almonds

1½ cups crushed walnuts

½ cup whole raw cashews

1 cup ground flaxseed

¼ cup raw cacao nibs

¼ cup unsweetened cocoa powder

⅛ teaspoon salt

¼ cup coconut oil

2 tablespoons granulated stevia

10 drops liquid stevia

1 teaspoon vanilla extract

1. Preheat oven to 300°F. Line a baking sheet with parchment paper.

2. Put nuts, flaxseed, cacao nibs, cocoa powder, and salt in a medium bowl and stir to combine.

3. In a small saucepan, melt coconut oil over low heat and stir in stevia and vanilla. Pour melted oil over nut mixture and toss to coat.

4. Spread nuts out on baking sheet and bake 15 minutes, stirring once halfway into cooking. Remove from oven and allow to cool completely.

Cauliflower Hash

This Cauliflower Hash complements poached eggs and some pan-fried turkey bacon perfectly.

INGREDIENTS | SERVES 2

1 tablespoon olive oil
3 cups chopped cauliflower
1 small yellow onion, peeled and diced
¼ teaspoon smoked paprika
¼ teaspoon salt
⅛ teaspoon ground black pepper
½ teaspoon garlic powder
1 teaspoon dried chives

1. Heat oil in a large skillet over medium-high heat and add cauliflower and onion. Cook until cauliflower is tender but not mushy—stirring only occasionally so that the cauliflower can brown, about 7 minutes.

2. Remove from heat, add spices and chives, and stir until combined.

3. Serve immediately.

The Versatile Cauliflower

One of the great things about cauliflower is that it's so versatile. Its natural flavor is so mild that it picks up the flavors of whatever spices you add to it very nicely.

Smoked Salmon–Wrapped Asparagus with Poached Eggs

After you try these smoked salmon–wrapped asparagus spears, you'll never want to go back to the traditional bacon-wrapped ones again.

INGREDIENTS | SERVES 2

8 medium asparagus spears, ends trimmed

1 tablespoon olive oil

1 teaspoon dried rosemary

1 teaspoon dried thyme

⅛ teaspoon salt

⅛ teaspoon ground black pepper

3 cups water

4 large eggs

2 ounces smoked salmon

1. Preheat oven to 400°F.

2. Line a baking sheet with foil and spread out asparagus spears. Drizzle with olive oil and sprinkle with rosemary, thyme, salt, and pepper.

3. Bake asparagus until slightly browned, about 10 minutes.

4. While asparagus is cooking, put water in a medium saucepan and bring to a boil over high heat. Reduce heat to medium-low and crack eggs into water. Cook until whites have set but yolks are still runny, about 3–4 minutes.

5. Remove asparagus from oven and wrap spears in smoked salmon. Place poached eggs on top. Serve immediately.

Breakfast Burrito

Ham makes a more than suitable replacement for a tortilla wrap in this Breakfast Burrito recipe. You can also use sliced turkey or roast beef in place of ham.

INGREDIENTS | SERVES 1

1 tablespoon olive oil

¼ cup chopped spinach

2 large eggs, lightly beaten

⅛ cup sliced black olives

2 slices sugar-free ham

¼ medium avocado, pitted, flesh removed, and sliced thinly

1. Heat olive oil in a medium skillet over medium heat. Add spinach and cook until wilted, about 3 minutes. Add eggs and scramble until cooked through, about 4 minutes. Remove from heat and stir in olives.

2. Lay ham slices flat and top each slice with half the egg mixture and half the sliced avocado.

3. Roll up like a burrito and secure with a toothpick. Serve immediately.

MD Stage 2 Lunch

Eggplant Pizza

To test an eggplant for ripeness, lightly press your finger on its skin. If your finger does not leave an imprint, the eggplant isn't ready. Smaller eggplants tend to be sweeter and generally contain fewer seeds than larger eggplants.

INGREDIENTS | SERVES 4

1 (½-pound) American eggplant
2¼ teaspoons salt, divided
1 tablespoon plus 2 teaspoons olive oil
2 teaspoons minced garlic
1½ teaspoons dried basil, divided
1½ teaspoons dried oregano, divided
2 cups peeled, diced tomatoes
¼ cup tomato sauce (no sugar added)
1 tablespoon tomato paste
¼ teaspoon ground black pepper
½ cup chopped fresh basil

Know Your Eggplants

There are over half a dozen different eggplant varieties. American—also called globe eggplant—is the most familiar to the average consumer. American eggplants are large, dark purple, and pear shaped.

1. Preheat oven to 375°F. Line a baking sheet with parchment paper.

2. Cut eggplant into ½"-thick slices and place slices on paper towels. Sprinkle both sides of eggplant slices with 2 teaspoons salt to help draw out any excess water.

3. While eggplant sits, heat 1 tablespoon olive oil in a medium skillet over medium heat. Add garlic and sauté until fragrant, about 3 minutes.

4. Add ½ teaspoon dried basil, ½ teaspoon oregano, diced tomatoes, tomato sauce, tomato paste, ¼ teaspoon salt, and pepper. Stir to combine and then reduce heat to low. Allow sauce to simmer until it thickens, about 30–45 minutes.

5. Wipe eggplant dry with paper towels to remove excess liquid and most of the salt. Arrange eggplant slices on the baking sheet.

6. Sprinkle remaining dried basil and oregano on eggplant slices, drizzle with remaining olive oil, and bake 20 minutes. Remove eggplant from oven, scoop sauce onto top of each slice, and sprinkle with fresh basil.

7. Switch oven to low broil and return eggplant to oven another 5–7 minutes or until sauce is slightly browned and bubbling. Allow to cool slightly before serving.

Baked Meatballs

Most grocery stores and butcher shops have meatloaf mixture—a combination of beef, veal, and pork—already ground for you, but if they don't, you can either buy them separately and mix them or choose your favorite of the three.

INGREDIENTS | SERVES 4

1 pound ground meatloaf meat mixture (beef, veal, and pork)

2 teaspoons garlic powder

1 teaspoon dried minced onion

½ teaspoon salt

¼ teaspoon ground black pepper

2 teaspoons dried chives

2 large eggs

1. Preheat oven to 375°F. Line a baking sheet with parchment paper.

2. Combine all ingredients in a mixing bowl and use your hands to mix everything together to make sure all ingredients are incorporated.

3. Roll meat mixture into 1½" meatballs and arrange on the baking sheet.

4. Bake 25 minutes or until meatballs are browned and completely cooked through.

Chicken and Egg Salad

This is a simple lunch that's packed with protein and healthy fats. Double the recipe and you'll have enough on hand for your lunch for the entire week.

INGREDIENTS | SERVES 4

2 hard-boiled large eggs, peeled and roughly chopped

1 (12.5-ounce) can shredded chicken breast

2 tablespoons Homemade Mayonnaise (see recipe in Chapter 10)

½ teaspoon seasoned salt

½ teaspoon dried minced onion

¼ teaspoon ground black pepper

2 tablespoons minced red onion

1 stalk celery, diced

4 cups chopped romaine lettuce

1. Place all ingredients except lettuce in a medium mixing bowl and mix until everything is thoroughly combined.

2. Scoop ¼ chicken mixture onto 1 cup romaine lettuce for each serving. Serve immediately.

Chicken Burgers

*For an added boost of healthy fats, throw some sliced avocado
on top of this chicken burger along with the salsa.*

INGREDIENTS | SERVES 4

1 pound ground chicken

1 clove garlic, minced

1 teaspoon dried minced onion

1 large egg

3 tablespoons chopped fresh parsley

½ teaspoon salt

¼ teaspoon chili powder

½ teaspoon ground cumin

1 teaspoon dried chives

2 teaspoons coconut aminos

2 tablespoons olive oil

4 large romaine lettuce leaves

½ cup salsa

1. Combine chicken, garlic, onion, egg, parsley, salt, chili powder, cumin, chives, and coconut aminos in a medium mixing bowl and use your hands to mix ingredients. Shape mixture into four patties.

2. Heat olive oil in a medium skillet over medium-high heat. Add burger patties to hot oil and cook 5–7 minutes on each side or until chicken is no longer pink and juices run clear.

3. Remove from heat and top each burger with lettuce and ⅛ cup salsa.

What Are Coconut Aminos?

Coconut aminos are made from the sap that comes out of the coconut blossoms of the coconut tree once it's tapped. Coconut aminos have a taste similar to soy sauce, but unlike soy sauce, they are an abundant source of amino acids, vitamins, and minerals.

Cucumber, Tomato, and Tuna Salad

You can swap out the tuna for canned shredded chicken or canned salmon for some variations on this simple lunchtime recipe.

INGREDIENTS | SERVES 2

1 medium cucumber, sliced thinly

1 medium tomato, sliced into
thin wedges

¼ medium red onion, peeled and cut
into rings

1 (5-ounce) can tuna packed in water

1½ tablespoons red wine vinegar

2 tablespoons olive oil

½ teaspoon coarse salt

¼ teaspoon coarse ground pepper

2 teaspoons chopped fresh parsley

1. Combine cucumber, tomato, red onion, and tuna in a medium mixing bowl and stir to combine.

2. In a small bowl, whisk together vinegar, olive oil, salt, pepper, and parsley. Pour oil mixture into cucumber mixture and toss to coat. Serve immediately.

Think about Your Tuna

When choosing a tuna, opt for one that is pole-caught and sustainable. Many big-name tuna companies use nets to catch their tuna, which unnecessarily puts other marine life in danger.

Lemon-Garlic Shrimp with Puréed Avocado

If you'd rather make this lemon-garlic shrimp on the stovetop, you can heat up some olive oil in a pan and sauté the shrimp just until it turns pink. Be careful not to overcook, which can make your shrimp chewy.

INGREDIENTS | SERVES 4

1 large avocado, pitted, flesh removed, and diced

1 teaspoon salt, divided

½ teaspoon ground black pepper

¼ teaspoon ground cumin

½ medium jalapeño pepper, seeded and minced

12 jumbo shrimp, deveined and peeled

2 teaspoons olive oil

1 clove garlic, minced

½ teaspoon lemon pepper

1. Put avocado, ½ teaspoon salt, black pepper, and cumin in a food processor and process until smooth. Stir in minced jalapeño.

2. Heat up grill. Thread three jumbo shrimp onto each of four skewers.

3. In a small bowl, whisk together olive oil, garlic, and lemon pepper. Brush oil mixture on shrimp. Grill shrimp 3 minutes on each side or until just pink. Serve with puréed avocado.

Shredded Chicken Greek Salad

Using a can of shredded chicken breast saves some time, but you can also grill up a couple of chicken breasts to serve on top of this salad instead.

INGREDIENTS | SERVES 2

¼ cup olive oil

2 tablespoons red wine vinegar

2 tablespoons apple cider vinegar

1 teaspoon dried oregano

½ teaspoon dried basil

¼ teaspoon salt

⅛ teaspoon ground black pepper

4 cups chopped romaine lettuce

¼ cup chopped red onion

1 medium cucumber, chopped

12 cherry tomatoes, cut in half

1 (12.5-ounce) can shredded chicken breast

½ cup kalamata olives

1. In a small bowl, whisk together oil, vinegars, oregano, basil, salt, and pepper. Set aside.

2. In a large bowl, combine lettuce, onion, cucumber, tomato, and chicken. Use two knives to chop salad and combine ingredients.

3. Add olives and dressing and toss to combine. Serve immediately.

The Magical ACV

Apple cider vinegar has been shown to improve insulin sensitivity during a high-carbohydrate meal by as much as 34 percent. Including apple cider vinegar in your daily diet can also significantly improve glucose and insulin responses to meals. Human studies also show that ACV can increase satiety and help you eat fewer calories during the day.

Mini Crab Cakes with Spicy Aioli

Don't let the fancy name of this lunch scare you away; making these crab cakes is surprisingly easy, and the end result is worth it.

INGREDIENTS | SERVES 2

1 (8-ounce) can jumbo lump blue crabmeat

2 large egg whites

¼ teaspoon red pepper flakes

1 teaspoon dried chives

¼ cup plus 1 tablespoon Homemade Mayonnaise (see recipe in Chapter 10)

2 teaspoons fresh lemon juice

4 cloves garlic, minced

1 teaspoon tomato paste

½ teaspoon smoked paprika

⅛ teaspoon cayenne pepper

1 tablespoon olive oil

1. Combine crab, egg whites, red pepper, chives, and 1 tablespoon mayonnaise in a large bowl and mix until combined. Form mixture into patties.

2. Put remaining mayonnaise, lemon juice, garlic, tomato paste, paprika, and cayenne in a food processor and process until smooth.

3. Heat olive oil in a medium skillet over medium heat and cook crab patties 10 minutes or until cakes are browned and heated through, flipping once.

4. Top crab cakes with aioli and serve immediately.

Succulent Crab

Crabmeat is considered a delicacy in some parts of the world because of its sweet taste and rich flavor. Crab is rich in protein and contains no carbohydrates. Crabmeat also contains high amounts of vitamin B_{12}, which contributes to proper brain and nervous system function.

Tuna and Artichoke Salad

You can generally find marinated artichoke hearts in the Italian section of your supermarket or in the aisle that also holds the pickles and olives.

INGREDIENTS | SERVES 2

2 (5-ounce) cans chunk light tuna in water

3 tablespoons Homemade Mayonnaise (see recipe in Chapter 10)

½ cup chopped marinated artichoke hearts

¼ cup chopped roasted red peppers

½ teaspoon seasoned salt

¼ teaspoon ground black pepper

4 cups mixed greens

1. Combine all ingredients except mixed greens in a large bowl and mix with a fork until all ingredients are combined.

2. Serve tuna salad over lettuce.

Start Eating Artichoke

Artichoke hearts aren't the most commonly consumed vegetable, but many think they should be. Artichokes are loaded with phytonutrients, like quercetin, rutin, gallic acid, and cynarin. These phytonutrients work together to protect against heart disease, cancer, liver disease, and diabetes.

Roast Beef and Turkey Lettuce Wraps

This quick recipe is perfect for when you have to make a lunch with only minutes to spare.
You can use any deli meat that doesn't contain added sugar or artificial ingredients.

INGREDIENTS | SERVES 2

4 large romaine lettuce leaves
4 slices (4 ounces) roast beef
4 slices (4 ounces) turkey
2 teaspoons yellow mustard
2 medium pickle spears, cut in half

1. Lay romaine leaves out flat and top each leaf with 1 slice roast beef and 1 slice turkey. Drizzle with ½ teaspoon yellow mustard and half a pickle spear.

2. Roll lettuce into wrap. Serve immediately.

Salmon with Dill Sauce

This basic recipe works well with any type of fish. Rotate between salmon,
cod, and sea bass if you're looking to switch things up.

INGREDIENTS | SERVES 4

¼ cup Homemade Mayonnaise (see recipe in Chapter 10)
1 tablespoon chopped fresh dill
2 teaspoons spicy brown mustard
1 teaspoon lemon juice
¼ teaspoon garlic salt
½ teaspoon prepared horseradish
4 (4-ounce) salmon fillets
1 teaspoon lemon pepper
1 teaspoon onion powder
4 slices lemon

1. Preheat oven to 350°F.

2. Combine mayonnaise, dill, mustard, lemon juice, garlic salt, and horseradish in a food processor and process until smooth.

3. Place salmon skin-side down on a foil-lined baking dish. Sprinkle lemon pepper and onion powder on top and top with lemon. Bake 20–25 minutes or until fish flakes easily with a fork.

4. Remove from oven and top with dill sauce.

Stuffed Peppers

The fire-roasted tomatoes in this recipe add some spice to the dish without being too hot. If you'd prefer to dial it back a bit, replace the fire-roasted tomatoes with regular diced tomatoes or chopped fresh tomatoes.

INGREDIENTS | SERVES 4

2 tablespoons olive oil

1 medium yellow onion, peeled and chopped

2 cloves garlic, minced

1 pound lean ground beef

1 teaspoon ground cumin

1 teaspoon chili powder

1 teaspoon smoked paprika

½ teaspoon garlic salt

¼ teaspoon ground black pepper

1 (14.5-ounce) can diced fire-roasted tomatoes

½ cup sliced black olives

4 large bell peppers (any color), tops cut off and seeded

1. Preheat oven to 350°F.

2. In a large skillet, heat olive oil over medium-high heat. Add onion and garlic and sauté until translucent, about 4 minutes.

3. Add beef and continue to cook. Add cumin, chili powder, paprika, garlic salt, and pepper and continue to cook until beef is no longer pink, about 7 minutes.

4. Add fire-roasted tomatoes and cook 5 more minutes or until some of the liquid has evaporated. Remove from heat and stir in black olives.

5. Place peppers cut-side up in a baking dish and fill each pepper with ¼ beef mixture. Bake 30 minutes or until peppers are softened and starting to brown. Serve immediately.

Shrimp Salad Wraps

Instead of romaine lettuce leaves, you may opt for Swiss chard leaves or cabbage leaves, which are a little tougher but may hold up better as a wrap.

INGREDIENTS | SERVES 4

¼ cup Homemade Mayonnaise (see recipe in Chapter 10)

1 tablespoon fresh lemon juice

1 teaspoon white vinegar

1 teaspoon celery salt

½ teaspoon dried minced onion

¼ teaspoon ground black pepper

1 pound frozen large shrimp, completely thawed and roughly chopped

½ cup finely chopped celery

3 tablespoons dried chives

8 large romaine lettuce leaves

1. In a small bowl, combine mayonnaise, lemon juice, vinegar, celery salt, onion, and pepper and whisk until combined.

2. In a large bowl, combine shrimp, chopped celery, and chives. Pour dressing over shrimp and toss to coat. Refrigerate 30 minutes.

3. After shrimp mixture is chilled, scoop into romaine leaves and serve immediately.

Salsa Chicken

This Salsa Chicken is a Mexican food lover's dream. It gives all the flavor of a plate of tacos without any of the metabolism-destroying ingredients.

INGREDIENTS | SERVES 4

1 tablespoon chili powder

1½ teaspoons ground cumin

1 teaspoon salt

1 teaspoon ground black pepper

½ teaspoon paprika

¼ teaspoon dried oregano

¼ teaspoon red pepper flakes

¼ teaspoon onion powder

¼ teaspoon garlic powder

4 (4-ounce) boneless skinless chicken breasts

1 cup salsa (no sugar added)

½ cup sliced black olives

Making Your Own Chili Powder

If you don't have premade chili powder at home, you can mix your own with several spices you probably already have on hand—paprika, oregano, cumin, garlic powder, onion powder, and cayenne pepper.

1. Preheat oven to 350°F.

2. Combine chili powder, cumin, salt, black pepper, paprika, oregano, red pepper flakes, onion powder, and garlic powder in a gallon-sized plastic bag and shake to combine.

3. Add chicken to bag and shake to completely coat with spice mixture.

4. Put chicken in a baking dish and top each breast with ¼ cup salsa. Bake 30 minutes or until chicken is no longer pink and juices run clear.

5. Remove from oven and top with sliced olives. Serve immediately.

Mediterranean Zoodles

This recipe also makes a wonderful cold zucchini salad. Instead of cooking the zucchini, mix all ingredients together and allow the mixture to sit in the refrigerator for 20 minutes before eating.

INGREDIENTS | SERVES 4

4 large zucchini, julienned or cut into spirals with a spiralizer

¼ cup plus 1 tablespoon olive oil

¾ cup cherry tomatoes, cut in half

¾ cup marinated artichoke hearts, roughly chopped

½ cup kalamata olives

½ large avocado, pitted, flesh removed, and diced

2 tablespoons fresh lemon juice

1 tablespoon white vinegar

2 cloves garlic, minced

½ teaspoon salt

¼ teaspoon ground black pepper

1. Set zucchini "noodles" aside on a paper towel and allow to "sweat" 5 minutes.

2. Heat 1 tablespoon olive oil in a medium skillet and add zucchini, tomatoes, artichoke, and olives. Sauté until zucchini just starts to soften, about 3 minutes.

3. Remove from heat and toss in avocado.

4. In a small bowl, whisk together remaining oil, lemon juice, vinegar, garlic, salt, and pepper. Pour dressing over zucchini mixture and toss to coat. Serve immediately.

Chicken and Bacon Casserole

This recipe is a completely balanced meal in and of itself—it has protein, green vegetables, and healthy fats in the form of coconut cream.

INGREDIENTS | SERVES 8

½ pound turkey bacon, roughly chopped

2 pounds boneless skinless chicken breasts, cubed

2 cups chopped broccoli

1 cup chicken broth

¼ cup coconut cream

3 tablespoons Dijon mustard

2 teaspoons Italian seasoning

½ teaspoon salt

¼ teaspoon ground black pepper

Not All Coconut Cream Is Created Equal

Many of the "coconut creams" sold in stores contain added sweeteners. You can get the same effect without any of the sugar by opening up a can of full-fat coconut milk, without shaking it, and spooning out the hard part that sits on top. This part of the milk is also called the coconut cream.

1. Preheat oven to 350°F.

2. Cook bacon in a large skillet over medium-high heat until cooked through, about 6 minutes. Add cubed chicken to pan and continue to cook until chicken is no longer pink, about 7–8 minutes. Remove from heat and stir in chopped broccoli.

3. In a medium bowl, combine broth, coconut cream, mustard, Italian seasoning, salt, and pepper. Pour mixture over chicken mixture and stir to combine.

4. Pour mixture into a 9" × 13" casserole dish and bake 30 minutes or until it starts to brown and get bubbly.

Spicy Shrimp Salad

The horseradish in this recipe gives this salad a delicious metabolism-boosting kick.

INGREDIENTS | SERVES 4

1 tablespoon olive oil

1 pound frozen cooked shrimp, thawed completely

½ teaspoon garlic powder

½ teaspoon onion powder

½ teaspoon chili powder

½ teaspoon paprika

½ teaspoon salt

¼ teaspoon ground black pepper

¼ cup avocado oil

1 tablespoon prepared horseradish

1 tablespoon spicy brown mustard

2 teaspoons white vinegar

8 cups shredded lettuce

1. Heat olive oil in a medium skillet over medium heat. Add cooked shrimp along with garlic powder, onion powder, chili powder, paprika, salt, and pepper. Stir to coat shrimp and heat through, about 3–4 minutes.

2. In a small bowl, combine avocado oil, horseradish, mustard, and vinegar and whisk until smooth.

3. Place cooked shrimp over lettuce and pour on dressing mixture. Toss to coat. Serve immediately.

A Lesson on Horseradish

Horseradish is a member of the Brassicaceae family, which makes it closely related to mustard, cabbage, broccoli, and wasabi. When the thick, white root of horseradish is sliced, the plant releases enzymes that break down a compound, called sinigrin, in the root. This releases the mustard oil, which gives horseradish its signature scent and flavor.

Salmon-Stuffed Zucchini Bites

For this recipe, you could also use sliced cucumber in place of the zucchini.
Both green vegetables are low in calories and high in water content.

INGREDIENTS | SERVES 2

2 medium zucchini

1 (6-ounce) can salmon

3 tablespoons Homemade Mayonnaise
(see recipe in Chapter 10)

½ teaspoon dry mustard

½ teaspoon salt

¼ teaspoon ground black pepper

2 tablespoons minced green onion

1 teaspoon chopped fresh dill

1. Cut zucchini into ½" slices and use a small spoon to scoop out a bowl in the center of each slice. Arrange on a serving tray.

2. In a medium bowl, combine remaining ingredients and stir with a fork until combined.

3. Scoop salmon mixture into holes in zucchini. Serve immediately.

A Low-Calorie Choice

Zucchini is the perfect addition to any meal because it's rich in nutrients but ultralow in calories. One cup of zucchini only has about 20 calories, which is about half that of the same size of other low-calorie green vegetables like broccoli.

Turkey and Hummus Lettuce Wraps

This recipe calls for prepared hummus, which you can buy at the store or easily make at home. If you choose to buy a store-bought version, read the labels and make sure there's no added sugar or artificial ingredients.

INGREDIENTS | SERVES 2

4 large leaves iceberg lettuce

4 tablespoons prepared hummus

8 slices (8 ounces) roasted turkey

1 medium cucumber, cut into matchsticks

½ cup alfalfa sprouts

½ large lemon

1. Lay iceberg lettuce leaves out and spread 1 tablespoon hummus on each leaf. Top hummus with 2 slices turkey and ¼ of the sliced cucumber and sprouts. Sprinkle with lemon juice.

2. Roll each lettuce wrap and secure with a toothpick. Serve immediately.

Homemade Hummus

Hummus is easy to make at home. All you need is a can of chickpeas, juice from 1 large lemon, ¼ cup tahini, 1 clove garlic, 2 tablespoons olive oil, 1 teaspoon salt, ½ teaspoon cumin, and 2 tablespoons water. Put all ingredients together in a food processor and process until smooth.

Tuna-Stuffed Eggs

You can try different variations of this recipe by replacing the tuna with canned salmon, canned chicken, or even lump crabmeat.

INGREDIENTS | SERVES 2

4 hard-boiled large eggs, peeled, halved, and yolks removed

4 ounces canned tuna

¼ cup Homemade Mayonnaise (see recipe in Chapter 10)

1 tablespoon dried chives

½ teaspoon celery salt

¼ teaspoon ground black pepper

¼ teaspoon smoked paprika

1. Add egg yolks, tuna, mayonnaise, chives, celery salt, and pepper into a medium bowl. Stir until combined.

2. Scoop yolk mixture into egg whites and sprinkle with paprika. Refrigerate 30–60 minutes before serving.

BLT Sushi Rolls

This recipe doesn't technically qualify as sushi since it doesn't contain any rice or fish, but you'll forget all that when you taste the bacon, lettuce, and tomato combination.

INGREDIENTS | SERVES 4

4 nori wraps

4 slices cooked turkey bacon

2 cups chopped romaine lettuce

2 small tomatoes, seeded and sliced into strips

½ large avocado, pitted, flesh removed, and sliced into strips

1 teaspoon cayenne pepper sauce

½ cup coconut aminos

1 tablespoon Homemade Mayonnaise (see recipe in Chapter 10)

1 teaspoon lime juice

1 teaspoon sesame oil

1. Lay nori wraps flat. At the edge of each wrap, stack 1 slice turkey bacon, ½ cup lettuce, ¼ of the tomato slices and ⅛ of the avocado. Drizzle ¼ teaspoon cayenne pepper sauce on top. Use a brush to wet the other edge of the seaweed wrap and roll. Cut each wrap into 6–8 slices (like sushi).

2. Combine coconut aminos, mayonnaise, lime juice, and sesame oil in a food processor and process until smooth.

3. Serve sushi rolls with dipping sauce.

Buffalo Chicken Lettuce Wraps

You can make this recipe even quicker by using canned shredded chicken in place of the chicken breasts. Since they're precooked, all you would have to do is toss the ingredients together then serve.

INGREDIENTS | SERVES 2

2 tablespoons olive oil

2 (4-ounce) boneless skinless chicken breasts, cooked and shredded

½ cup hot sauce

½ teaspoon salt

¼ teaspoon ground black pepper

1 stalk celery, finely chopped

4 large iceberg lettuce leaves

½ cup Homemade Ranch Dressing (see recipe in Chapter 10)

1. Heat olive oil in a medium skillet over medium heat. Add shredded chicken along with hot sauce, salt, and pepper. Cook until heated through.

2. Remove from heat and toss in chopped celery.

3. Scoop chicken into each lettuce leaf and drizzle ⅛ cup ranch dressing on top of each.

4. Roll lettuce wrap and secure with a toothpick. Serve immediately.

Spicy Chickpea Salad

Make this recipe vegetarian-friendly by omitting the salmon. The chickpeas will provide enough protein to keep you full until your next snack.

INGREDIENTS | SERVES 2

1 (5-ounce) can salmon, drained

1 (15-ounce) can chickpeas, drained and rinsed

2 stalks celery, finely chopped

1 medium shallot, peeled and minced

1 clove garlic, minced

1 large cucumber, diced

1 cup cherry tomatoes, halved

¼ cup olive oil

Juice from ½ large lemon

½ tablespoon apple cider vinegar

½ tablespoon red wine vinegar

1 teaspoon chopped fresh parsley

¼ teaspoon ground black pepper

¼ teaspoon ground cumin

¼ teaspoon red pepper flakes

1. In a large bowl, combine salmon, chickpeas, celery, shallot, garlic, cucumber, and tomatoes and mix until evenly incorporated.

2. In a small bowl, whisk together remaining ingredients.

3. Pour dressing over chickpea mixture and toss to coat. Refrigerate 1 hour before serving.

Onions versus Shallots

Like onions and garlic, shallots belong to the *Allium* genus. They have a richer and sweeter flavor than onions and tend to incorporate into recipes, especially sauces, a little more easily. They are more potent than onions, so you only need about half the amount. They pair especially well with chicken and fish.

Chicken Caesar Lettuce Wraps

The anchovies in this recipe are marked as optional, but they really add a depth of flavor to the Caesar dressing that can't be beat. Most Caesar dressings contain anchovies anyway, but you might just not know it!

INGREDIENTS | SERVES 4

¼ cup canned chickpeas, drained and rinsed

2 tablespoons raw cashews

3 tablespoons fresh lemon juice

¼ cup olive oil

¼ cup avocado oil

1 tablespoon tahini

1 teaspoon coconut aminos

½ teaspoon minced garlic

½ teaspoon dry mustard

¼ teaspoon ground black pepper

2 canned anchovies (optional)

1 (12-ounce) can shredded chicken breast

½ medium avocado, pitted, flesh removed, and diced

4 cups shredded romaine lettuce

4 large leaves romaine lettuce

1. Combine chickpeas, cashews, lemon juice, oils, tahini, coconut aminos, garlic, mustard, pepper, and anchovies in a food processor. Process until smooth.

2. In a large bowl, combine chicken, avocado, and shredded lettuce. Pour dressing over salad mixture and toss to combine.

3. Scoop dressed salad equally into each large lettuce leaf. Roll up like a wrap. Secure with a toothpick and serve immediately.

Good Things Come in Small Packages

Anchovies may be tiny, but don't write them off just because of their size. Anchovies are packed with just as much omega-3 fatty acids as salmon and twice that of whitefish, like halibut. Unlike other fish, anchovies are extremely low in mercury and other potential toxins. They are also one of the most sustainable options because they are not overfished.

Niçoise Salad

*A traditional niçoise salad contains potatoes, but you won't even miss
them when you try this low-carbohydrate, Stage 2 version.*

INGREDIENTS | SERVES 2

4 cups water
¾ pound green beans, washed and trimmed
1 cup halved cherry tomatoes
¾ cup kalamata olives, divided
4 cups mixed greens
3 hard-boiled large eggs, peeled and roughly chopped
2 (5.5-ounce) cans Italian tuna
1 tablespoon minced shallot
3 tablespoons red wine vinegar
¼ cup avocado oil
2 tablespoons chopped fresh basil
1 tablespoon Dijon mustard
¼ teaspoon ground black pepper

1. Bring water to a boil in a medium saucepan over medium-high heat and add green beans. Cook 2–4 minutes or until beans are tender but still crispy. Drain and allow to cool, then cut into thirds.

2. Combine beans, cherry tomatoes, ½ cup olives, greens, eggs, and tuna in a medium bowl and mix until evenly incorporated.

3. Remove the pits from the remaining ¼ cup olives and combine pitted olives with the remaining ingredients in a food processor. Process until smooth.

4. Pour dressing over salad mixture and toss to combine.

CHAPTER 9

MD Stage 2 Dinner

Slow Cooker Pulled Pork Chili

*After cooking this chili for 8 hours, shred the pork with two forks
and stir it up to incorporate the flavors into it.*

INGREDIENTS | SERVES 8

2 tablespoons smoked paprika

2 tablespoons garlic powder

1 tablespoon dried minced onion

1 tablespoon ground cumin

1 teaspoon cayenne pepper

1 teaspoon red pepper flakes

½ teaspoon dried oregano

1 teaspoon salt

¾ teaspoon ground black pepper

1 (2-pound) pork roast, fat trimmed

1 large yellow onion, peeled and diced

2 medium red bell peppers, seeded and diced

1 (14.5-ounce) can fire-roasted tomatoes

1 (14.5-ounce) can petite diced tomatoes

1 (14-ounce) can tomato sauce

3 tablespoons tomato paste

1. In a small bowl, combine paprika, garlic powder, onion, cumin, cayenne, red pepper flakes, oregano, salt, and black pepper.

2. Rub spice mixture all over pork roast, making sure to get it in every crevice. Refrigerate 4 hours or overnight.

3. Place roast in a slow cooker and add remaining ingredients, stirring to combine.

4. Cook on low 8 hours or until pork shreds easily with a fork.

Eggplant Lasagna

Thin slices of eggplant take the place of carbohydrate-laden noodles in this lasagna dish. The flavor is so developed, you won't even miss the noodles or the cheese.

INGREDIENTS | SERVES 8

2 tablespoons olive oil

1 small yellow onion, peeled and diced

4 cloves garlic, minced

1 pound ground beef

½ cup sliced mushrooms

2 (28-ounce) cans crushed tomatoes (no sugar added)

1 (14-ounce) can tomato sauce (no sugar added)

¼ cup extra-virgin olive oil

¼ cup red wine vinegar

2 tablespoons Italian seasoning

¼ cup chopped fresh parsley

¾ teaspoon salt

½ teaspoon ground black pepper

2 large American eggplants

Consider a Mandolin

The easiest way to slice the eggplant into long, thin strips is to use a mandolin slicer. A mandolin slicer will not only get the slices thinner than you may be able to with a knife, but it will also make them more uniform. If you do use a mandolin, make sure to use the guard when slicing to avoiding cutting your fingers.

1. Preheat oven to 350°F.

2. Heat olive oil in a large stockpot over medium-high heat. Add onion and garlic and sauté until browned, about 5 minutes. Add beef and cook until no longer pink. Add mushrooms and cook until softened, about 4 minutes.

3. Add crushed tomatoes, tomato sauce, extra-virgin olive oil, red wine vinegar, and seasonings. Stir and allow to come to a simmer.

4. Simmer 45 minutes, stirring occasionally.

5. While sauce is cooking, slice eggplant into long, thin strips that resemble lasagna noodles.

6. Layer the bottom of a 9" × 13" baking dish with eggplant and top with 2 cups sauce mixture. Layer more eggplant on top of sauce and then add 2 more cups sauce. Continue layering until eggplant and sauce are gone.

7. Bake in oven 1 hour. Allow to cool before serving.

Blackened Salmon

Blackening is a cooking technique most often associated with Cajun dishes.
The technique works extremely well with fish and chicken.

INGREDIENTS | SERVES 2

½ teaspoon garlic powder
½ teaspoon onion powder
2 teaspoons smoked paprika
¼ teaspoon ground cumin
⅛ teaspoon cayenne pepper
½ teaspoon salt
¼ teaspoon ground black pepper
2 (6-ounce) salmon fillets
1 tablespoon olive oil

1. Preheat oven to 400°F.

2. Combine garlic powder, onion powder, paprika, cumin, cayenne, salt, and black pepper in a small bowl.

3. Rub spice mixture over salmon, covering all areas.

4. Heat olive oil in a large cast-iron skillet over medium-high heat. Cook salmon 2 minutes on each side and then transfer entire skillet to the preheated oven. Bake 10–15 more minutes or until fish flakes easily with a fork.

Farm-Raised versus Wild-Caught Salmon

Choosing wild-caught salmon over farm-raised salmon is your best bet for many reasons. Wild-caught salmon contains more calcium, iron, and potassium and has almost one-third fewer calories than farm-raised. Farm-raised salmon is also often injected with an artificial coloring to make it appear pinker.

Pork Roast with Vegetables

Make sure you add the vegetables to this pork roast well into the cooking time. If you add them in the beginning, you'll end up with charred vegetables by the time the roast is fully cooked.

INGREDIENTS | SERVES 6

2 cloves garlic, minced

4 teaspoons dried rosemary

2 teaspoons dried marjoram

1 teaspoon ground coriander

½ teaspoon ground sage

1 teaspoon salt, divided

¼ teaspoon ground black pepper

1 (2-pound) boneless pork loin

1 small head broccoli, cut into florets

1 small head cauliflower, cut into florets

1 tablespoon olive oil

1. Preheat oven to 325°F.

2. In a small bowl, combine garlic, rosemary, marjoram, coriander, sage, ½ teaspoon salt, and pepper. Rub spice mixture all over pork.

3. Place pork in a roasting pan, cover, and bake 1 hour. Remove cover and bake another 15 minutes.

4. While pork is cooking, place broccoli and cauliflower in a large bowl, toss in olive oil, and sprinkle with remaining salt. After 1 hour and 15 minutes, add vegetables to roasting pan around pork and cook an additional 30–45 minutes or until vegetables are tender and pork is cooked through.

Lettuce Wrap Tacos

Corn and flour tortillas will become a thing of the past after you try these lettuce-wrapped tacos. They fill you up without spiking your blood sugar.

INGREDIENTS | SERVES 4

1 tablespoon chili powder

1½ teaspoons ground cumin

1 teaspoon salt

1 teaspoon ground black pepper

½ teaspoon paprika

¼ teaspoon red pepper flakes

¼ teaspoon dried oregano

¼ teaspoon garlic powder

¼ teaspoon onion powder

1 pound ground turkey

8 large iceberg lettuce leaves

1 cup salsa

2 tablespoons finely minced red onion

½ cup sliced black olives

½ large avocado, pitted, flesh removed, and sliced thinly

¼ cup chopped cilantro

1. Combine all spices in a small bowl.

2. Heat a medium skillet over medium heat and start to cook ground turkey. When meat is slightly browned, about 4 minutes, add spice mixture and stir to combine. Continue cooking turkey until no longer pink.

3. Divide meat evenly between lettuce leaves. Top each taco with salsa, minced onion, black olives, avocado, and cilantro.

Cilantro Cleaning Tip

Like spinach, cilantro is known for being really sandy. The easiest way to wash cilantro is to fill up a bowl with cold water, then dunk the cilantro leaves in the bowl while holding onto the stems. Swish the cilantro around in the water and then remove the leaves and shake the excess water off.

Slow Cooker Balsamic Chicken

For this recipe, choose a balsamic vinegar without any added sulfites. Sulfites that occur naturally are okay.

INGREDIENTS | SERVES 4

4 (4-ounce) boneless skinless chicken breasts

2 tablespoons olive oil

½ teaspoon dried oregano

½ teaspoon dried basil

½ teaspoon dried parsley

½ teaspoon dried thyme

½ teaspoon dried rosemary

1 teaspoon garlic powder

1 teaspoon salt

¼ teaspoon ground black pepper

1 medium yellow onion, peeled and roughly chopped

5 cloves garlic, minced

2 (14.5-ounce) cans petite diced tomatoes

1 (15-ounce) can tomato sauce

1 cup chicken broth

½ cup balsamic vinegar

1. Place chicken in the bottom of a slow cooker. Drizzle with olive oil.

2. Sprinkle seasonings directly on top of chicken, then cover with onion and garlic.

3. Pour remaining ingredients on top and cook on low 6–8 hours.

Pesto Zucchini "Pasta"

You can make this dinner vegetarian-friendly by omitting the turkey bacon and upping the protein by adding some rinsed chickpeas.

INGREDIENTS | SERVES 4

4 medium zucchini, julienned or cut into spirals with a spiralizer

1 teaspoon salt, divided

1 cup packed fresh basil leaves

1 clove garlic

⅛ cup pine nuts

5 tablespoons olive oil, divided

¼ teaspoon ground black pepper

2 cups broccoli florets

8 slices cooked turkey bacon, crumbled

¼ cup chopped green onions

The Relaxation Mineral

Just ½ cup pine nuts provides nearly half of the magnesium you need for an entire day. Most Americans are deficient in this mineral, which is often referred to as the relaxation mineral because it helps calm the nervous system and muscles.

1. Set zucchini in a strainer and sprinkle ½ teaspoon salt on top. Place strainer over a sink and allow excess water to drain out.

2. Combine basil, garlic, pine nuts, 3 tablespoons olive oil, remaining salt, and pepper in a food processor and process until smooth to make a pesto.

3. Heat up remaining 2 tablespoons olive oil in a medium skillet over medium-high heat. Add broccoli florets and cook until tender but still crisp, about 7 minutes.

4. Add drained zucchini and continue to cook until zucchini softens but still has a crunch, about 4 minutes.

5. Add bacon, green onions, and pesto and toss to combine. Continue cooking 1 more minute or until just heated through. Serve immediately.

Portobello Burgers

Mushrooms are porous, so you should never wash them with water. Instead, wipe them down with a dry paper towel before preparing them for cooking.

INGREDIENTS | SERVES 2

½ pound lean ground beef

1 teaspoon minced dried onion

½ teaspoon salt

¼ teaspoon plus ⅛ teaspoon ground black pepper

2 tablespoons olive oil

3 tablespoons balsamic vinegar

4 portobello mushroom caps

2 slices tomato

2 romaine lettuce leaves

¼ teaspoon coarse sea salt

The Sunshine Vitamin

Mushrooms are the only fruit or vegetable source of vitamin D, which many Americans are deficient in. Like humans, mushrooms can synthesize vitamin D when exposed to the sun.

1. In a large mixing bowl, combine beef, onion, salt, and ¼ teaspoon pepper. Form mixture into burger patties.

2. Heat up grill to medium-high heat. While grill is heating, combine olive oil and balsamic vinegar in a small bowl and brush mixture on mushroom caps.

3. Put burger patties on the grill and cook until desired doneness, about 5 minutes on each side. Remove burgers from grill and set aside.

4. Place mushrooms on grill stem-side down and cook 5 minutes. Flip mushrooms over and grill another 3 minutes. Remove mushrooms from grill, place a beef patty on top of a mushroom cap, top it with 1 slice tomato and 1 lettuce leaf, and then sprinkle coarse salt and remaining ⅛ teaspoon pepper on top. Cover with remaining mushroom cap. Serve immediately.

Chicken Curry

The term "curry" describes dishes that are based on South Asian cuisine. Traditional curry contains a mixture of turmeric, coriander, and cumin, which pair nicely with coconut.

INGREDIENTS | SERVES 4

2 tablespoons olive oil

4 (4-ounce) boneless skinless chicken breasts, cut into strips

1 teaspoon ground cumin

½ teaspoon ground ginger

½ teaspoon ground coriander

½ teaspoon ground turmeric

¼ teaspoon red pepper flakes

⅛ teaspoon ground cinnamon

2 teaspoons minced garlic

½ cup chicken broth

⅓ cup full-fat canned coconut milk

1. Heat olive oil in a large skillet over medium heat. Add chicken, spices, and garlic and cook until chicken is no longer pink, about 6 minutes.

2. Turn heat to high, add broth, and allow to come to a boil. Reduce heat to low and allow to simmer 5 minutes.

3. Slowly stir in coconut milk and allow to heat through, about 2 minutes. Serve immediately.

Canned versus Boxed Coconut Milk

The full-fat coconut milk you can get in the can is worlds apart from the processed stuff that comes in a box. Most boxed milks are full of preservatives and additives that increase their shelf life. They're also very thin since they're not 100 percent real coconut milk. Canned coconut milk contains very little additives—if any—and has a thick, rich consistency similar to that of heavy cream.

Coconut Shrimp

If you want to kick this Coconut Shrimp up a notch, add some cayenne pepper to the coconut mixture before coating the shrimp.

INGREDIENTS | SERVES 4

1 cup dried unsweetened coconut flakes
½ teaspoon salt
¼ teaspoon ground black pepper
1 large egg
1 pound medium shrimp, peeled and deveined
1 tablespoon olive oil

1. Combine coconut, salt, and pepper in a small bowl. In a separate bowl, lightly beat egg.

2. Dip each shrimp into egg and then coat with coconut mixture.

3. Heat olive oil in a medium skillet over medium-high heat. Put prepared shrimp in the skillet in batches, cooking 2–3 minutes on each side or until coconut is slightly browned and shrimp turns pink.

4. Serve immediately.

Roasted Chicken

Chicken and vegetables tend to be a staple "diet" food, but that doesn't mean they have to be boring and tasteless. Once you try this Roasted Chicken, it will become part of your regular menu.

INGREDIENTS | SERVES 8

1 (3-pound) whole roasting chicken
2 tablespoons olive oil
1 teaspoon dried thyme
2 teaspoons dried rosemary
2 teaspoons paprika
½ teaspoon salt
2 cups broccoli florets
2 cups cauliflower florets
2 cups chopped zucchini
3 teaspoons lemon pepper

Reduce Cooking Time

If you want to reduce the cooking time for this dish, you can cut the chicken apart into smaller pieces with kitchen scissors and then toss each piece in the spices to make sure they're fairly evenly coated.

1. Preheat oven to 350°F.

2. Put chicken in a roasting pan and rub with olive oil. Sprinkle, thyme, rosemary, paprika, and salt on chicken.

3. In a medium bowl, combine broccoli, cauliflower, and zucchini. Add lemon pepper and toss to coat. Arrange vegetables around chicken.

4. Bake 1 hour or until chicken reaches an internal temperature of 165°F.

5. Remove from heat and allow to cool slightly before serving.

Stuffed Portobello Mushrooms

Make this dish vegetarian by swapping the chicken breasts for some beans and extra vegetables, like broccoli and olives.

INGREDIENTS | SERVES 4

2 tablespoons olive oil, divided
6 ounces boneless skinless chicken breasts, cubed
1 tablespoon dried Italian seasoning
½ teaspoon salt
¼ teaspoon ground black pepper
2 cups chopped spinach
4 portobello mushroom caps
½ teaspoon garlic salt

Looking for Freshness

When choosing portobello mushrooms, look for firm mushrooms that are free of bruises and any shriveling. Any sliminess on the surface of the mushroom indicates that it is starting to spoil. The presence of a light layer of fuzz on a mushroom is a good sign—it indicates that the mushroom hasn't been handled much.

1. Preheat oven to broil.

2. While oven is preheating, heat 1 tablespoon olive oil in a medium skillet over medium-high heat. Add chicken, Italian seasoning, salt, and pepper and cook until chicken is no longer pink, about 6 minutes. Add spinach and cook until spinach wilts, about 3 more minutes.

3. Remove chicken mixture from heat and chop into small pieces.

4. Brush mushroom caps with remaining olive oil and sprinkle with garlic salt. Put mushroom caps on a baking sheet cap-side down and broil 3 minutes on each side.

5. Remove mushrooms from oven and stuff with chicken and spinach mixture. Return to the broiler 1 minute. Serve immediately.

Teriyaki Salmon

The term "teriyaki" traditionally refers to meat or fish that's been marinated in soy sauce and then grilled. Soy is out for the duration of this program, but you can reap the same flavor, with more benefits, by using coconut aminos instead.

INGREDIENTS | SERVES 2

¼ cup coconut aminos
1 cup water
½ teaspoon ground ginger
¼ teaspoon garlic powder
¾ teaspoon granulated stevia
2 (6-ounce) salmon fillets
1 tablespoon olive oil
2 teaspoons sesame seeds

1. Combine coconut aminos, water, ginger, garlic, and stevia in a medium bowl and whisk to combine.

2. Place salmon in marinade and marinate in the refrigerator 30 minutes.

3. Heat olive oil in a medium skillet over medium heat. Remove salmon from marinade and cook 5 minutes on each side or until salmon flakes easily with a fork.

4. Remove from heat and sprinkle with sesame seeds before serving.

Open Sesame

Sesame seeds don't get a lot of attention, but they're one of the oldest cultivated plants in the world. In ancient Egypt, the seeds were even one of the most popularly used medicines due to their nutritional value. Sesame seeds contain two unique compounds, sesamin and sesamolin, that are a type of fiber called lignans. Lignans have a cholesterol-lowering effect and may help prevent high blood pressure.

Chicken and Vegetable Kebabs

Marinating the chicken before cooking allows the flavors to really develop. If you can let the chicken sit in the marinade longer than 30 minutes, you'll get a stronger flavor and more tender chicken.

INGREDIENTS | SERVES 4

¼ cup olive oil

1 tablespoon fresh lemon juice

1 tablespoon apple cider vinegar

1 clove garlic, minced

½ teaspoon salt

¼ teaspoon ground black pepper

1 pound boneless skinless chicken breasts, cut into cubes

16 whole white mushrooms

1 large zucchini, cut into large chunks

1 large yellow summer squash, cut into large chunks

1. Combine olive oil, lemon juice, vinegar, garlic, salt, and pepper in a large gallon-sized plastic bag. Put chicken in bag, seal tightly, and refrigerate 30 minutes.

2. Preheat grill to medium heat. While grill is preheating, build eight skewers by alternating chicken with vegetables.

3. Grill 5–7 minutes on each side or until chicken is no longer pink and vegetables are tender but still crisp.

Baked Lemon Cod

Lemon and cod go together like spaghetti and meatballs. Up the lemon flavor by using the juice from one whole fresh lemon instead of just the half.

INGREDIENTS | SERVES 2

2 (6-ounce) cod fillets

1 tablespoon olive oil

2 teaspoons lemon pepper

2 teaspoons dried parsley

2 cloves garlic, minced

Juice from ½ large lemon

4 thin lemon slices

1. Preheat oven to 350°F.

2. Place cod fillets on a baking sheet lined with parchment paper. Rub olive oil on top of fish, then sprinkle with lemon pepper, dried parsley, and garlic.

3. Squeeze fresh lemon over fish and lay 2 lemon slices over each fillet.

4. Bake 15–20 minutes or until fish flakes easily with a fork.

Thai Chicken Tacos

Many Thai dishes contain peanuts and peanut sauces, but since peanuts are out on this program, this dish calls for SunButter—a brand of sunflower spread. SunButter is similar to peanut butter in taste and texture.

INGREDIENTS | SERVES 4

¼ cup plus 2 tablespoons coconut aminos

3 tablespoons freshly grated ginger, divided

Juice from ½ large lime

¼ teaspoon red pepper flakes

3 tablespoons toasted sesame seed oil, divided

4 (4-ounce) boneless skinless chicken breasts, cubed

2 tablespoons SunButter No Sugar Added

½ teaspoon ground cardamom

½ teaspoon ground turmeric

2 teaspoons full-fat coconut milk

1 tablespoon olive oil

8 green cabbage leaves

½ cup chopped roasted red peppers

½ cup bean sprouts

1. Combine ¼ cup coconut aminos, 1 tablespoon ginger, lime juice, red pepper flakes, and 2 tablespoons sesame oil in a plastic gallon-sized bag. Add chicken and marinate in refrigerator at least 4 hours.

2. Combine SunButter, remaining coconut aminos, remaining ginger, remaining sesame oil, cardamom, turmeric, and coconut milk in a food processor and process until smooth. Set aside.

3. Heat olive oil in a medium skillet over medium heat and add chicken. Cook until chicken is no longer pink, about 8 minutes.

4. Arrange cabbage leaves to form a cup. Scoop chicken into each cup, then top with roasted red peppers, sprouts, and sauce. Serve immediately.

Make Your Own!

Many commercial varieties of sunflower spread contain added sweetener since sunflower seeds don't have much natural sweeteners. You can easily make your own at home instead. Toast 2 cups of sunflower seeds in a dry skillet for about 4 minutes, stirring constantly. Add toasted sunflower seeds to a food processor and process for 10 minutes or until seeds start to break down and form a paste. When this happens, drizzle a teaspoon or two of sunflower seed oil in and keep processing. Eventually, it will turn into sunflower spread—just be patient!

Stuffed Filet Mignon

If you thought crab-stuffed filet mignon was only a treat you'd get to indulge in when going out to a five-star restaurant for a special occasion, think again.

INGREDIENTS | SERVES 2

2 (5-ounce) filet mignon medallions

½ cup lump blue crabmeat

1 tablespoon Homemade Mayonnaise (see recipe in Chapter 10)

1 tablespoon dried chives

½ teaspoon garlic salt

½ teaspoon salt

¼ teaspoon ground black pepper

1. Preheat oven broiler to low. Cut a slit in the side of each medallion to create a pocket.

2. In a medium bowl, combine crabmeat, mayonnaise, chives, and garlic salt. Stuff half the mixture into each medallion. Sprinkle medallions with salt and pepper.

3. Transfer medallions to a baking dish and broil on each side 6–7 minutes or until medallions reach desired level of doneness. Allow to sit 5 minutes before serving.

Chicken Sausage with Peppers and Onions

You can choose any variety of chicken sausage for this recipe—as long as it doesn't contain any added sugar—but the Italian sausage version pairs exceptionally well with the peppers and onions.

INGREDIENTS | SERVES 4

1 tablespoon olive oil

1 large yellow onion, peeled and sliced

1 medium red bell pepper, seeded and sliced

1 medium green bell pepper, seeded and sliced

3 cloves garlic, minced

½ teaspoon salt

½ teaspoon ground black pepper

1 teaspoon dried parsley

4 chicken sausages (no sugar added), cut into ¼"-thick coins

1. Heat olive oil in a medium skillet over medium-high heat. Add onion and cook 4 minutes. Add peppers, garlic, salt, black pepper, and parsley and continue to cook until peppers start to soften, about 5 more minutes.

2. Add chicken to onion and pepper mixture. Cook until chicken is browned on all sides and onion and peppers start to caramelize, about 7 minutes.

Fish Tacos

You can turn these Fish Tacos into a fish salad by chopping up the romaine lettuce, setting the fish on top, and using the dill sauce as a dressing.

INGREDIENTS | SERVES 4

1 clove garlic, minced

½ teaspoon ground cumin

½ teaspoon chili powder

1 pound cod

2 medium limes

1 tablespoon plus 1 teaspoon olive oil

½ small head red cabbage

½ medium onion, peeled and sliced thinly

3 tablespoons chopped fresh cilantro

¼ cup Homemade Mayonnaise (see recipe in Chapter 10)

1½ teaspoons lemon juice

1 tablespoon chopped fresh dill

¼ teaspoon garlic powder

⅛ teaspoon salt

⅛ teaspoon ground black pepper

1 teaspoon minced jalapeño pepper

8 large romaine lettuce leaves

1. In a small bowl, combine garlic, cumin, and chili powder. Coat cod with the mixture. Place cod in baking dish and squeeze the juice from 1 lime on top. Drizzle on 1 tablespoon olive oil and allow to marinate in the refrigerator 15 minutes.

2. While fish is marinating, preheat the grill to medium-high heat. Remove fish from marinade and grill 3 minutes on each side or until fish flakes easily with a fork. Set aside.

3. Roughly chop cabbage and put it in a medium bowl with onion and cilantro. Squeeze juice from remaining lime on top and add remaining olive oil. Set aside.

4. Combine mayonnaise, lemon juice, dill, garlic powder, salt, and pepper in a food processor and process until smooth. Stir in minced jalapeño.

5. Lay out each lettuce leaf and top with fish, then cabbage mixture, then dill sauce. Serve immediately.

Dill for Digestion

The essential oils present in dill help stimulate digestion and activate the secretion of bile and other juices that aid in the digestive process. These essential oils also stimulate peristalsis, the muscular contractions that physically move partially digested food through your digestive tract.

Slow Cooker Chicken Chili

If the liquid in this chili evaporates while cooking, add some more chicken broth until it reaches your desired consistency.

INGREDIENTS | SERVES 4

1 pound boneless skinless chicken breasts

1 medium red bell pepper, seeded and diced

1 medium yellow bell pepper, seeded and diced

1 medium jalapeño pepper, seeded and minced

1 medium yellow onion, peeled and diced

2 cloves garlic, minced

2 cups chicken broth

2 teaspoons chili powder

1 teaspoon ground cumin

1 teaspoon dried minced onion

1 teaspoon dried parsley

1 teaspoon salt

½ teaspoon ground black pepper

¼ cup chopped cilantro (optional)

1. Add all ingredients except cilantro to the slow cooker and stir to combine.

2. Cook on low 6–8 hours. Remove chicken and shred with a fork. Return to the slow cooker and stir to combine.

3. Top with cilantro if desired before serving.

CHAPTER 10

MD Stage 2 Snacks and Sides

Mediterranean Tomato Salad

If you don't have apple cider vinegar on hand, you can use white vinegar or red wine vinegar instead.

INGREDIENTS | SERVES 4

2 large tomatoes, seeded and diced

1 large cucumber, diced

¼ cup finely chopped red onion

¼ cup chopped mint

½ teaspoon salt

¼ cup apple cider vinegar

1 teaspoon granulated stevia

1½ tablespoons olive oil

½ cup kalamata olives

1. Combine all ingredients in a large bowl and toss to combine.

2. Refrigerate 1 hour before serving.

Protect Your Heart with Olives

Kalamata olives hold a place of prominence on the dinner table in Mediterranean regions around the world—and for good reason. Olives are most often praised for their high content of oleic acid—a mono-unsaturated fat that can help prevent heart disease—but they also contain antioxidant phenols that help thin the blood and dilate the blood vessels, ensuring proper flow of nutrients through the body.

Spicy Roast Beef Wraps

These Spicy Roast Beef Wraps are the perfect on-the-go snack. They're easy to throw together and travel with. Throw a handful of spinach in each wrap to add some green and boost the micronutrient content.

INGREDIENTS | SERVES 2

4 slices (4 ounces) roast beef

2 tablespoons Dijon mustard

2 teaspoons minced pickled jalapeños

1. Lay roast beef slices flat and spread ½ tablespoon mustard on each slice. Sprinkle ½ teaspoon jalapeños on top.

2. Roll and secure with a toothpick. Serve immediately.

Stuffed Mushrooms

If you don't have almond meal on hand, but you have some raw almonds, you can quickly make your own by throwing some almonds into a food processor and processing until the consistency reaches that of coarse sand.

INGREDIENTS | SERVES 5

10 whole button mushrooms

1 tablespoon olive oil

½ medium yellow onion, peeled and diced

1 clove garlic, minced

½ pound Italian sausage, casings removed

¼ cup almond meal

¼ teaspoon onion powder

¼ teaspoon ground black pepper

⅛ teaspoon cayenne pepper

Almond Flour versus Almond Meal

Almond flour and almond meal are both made from ground almonds, but they do have a couple of subtle differences. Almond flour is generally made from blanched almonds, which have no skin, and ground into a fine consistency. Almond meal is typically made from almonds that still have their skin and is a coarser grind.

1. Preheat oven to 350°F. Line a baking sheet with parchment paper.

2. Remove stems from mushrooms and chop stems into small pieces.

3. Heat olive oil in a medium skillet over medium heat. Add onion and garlic and sauté until softened, about 5 minutes. Add chopped mushroom stems and cook until softened, about 4 more minutes.

4. Add sausage and remaining ingredients and cook until sausage is no longer pink, about 5–7 minutes.

5. Fill each mushroom cap with stuffing and arrange stuffed-side up on the baking sheet. Bake 20–25 minutes or until stuffing and mushrooms are browned.

Homemade Ranch Dressing

This dressing isn't just for salads—use it as a sauce for your fish or chicken entrées or as a dip for some freshly cut vegetables. You can adjust the consistency by adding more or less coconut cream.

INGREDIENTS | MAKES 1½ CUPS (12 SERVINGS)

1 cup Homemade Mayonnaise (see recipe in this chapter)
½ cup coconut cream
½ teaspoon white vinegar
¼ cup chopped fresh parsley
2 tablespoons chopped fresh dill
½ teaspoon dried chives
¼ teaspoon garlic powder
¼ teaspoon onion powder
⅛ teaspoon salt
⅛ teaspoon ground black pepper

1. Put all ingredients in a medium mixing bowl and whisk until smooth.

2. Cover and refrigerate at least 30 minutes before serving.

Broccoli Slaw

If you can't find prepackaged broccoli slaw, you can make your own by passing raw broccoli florets through the shredding attachment of a food processor. You can also substitute the prepackaged broccoli slaw with regular dry, bagged coleslaw.

INGREDIENTS | SERVES 4

¼ cup Homemade Mayonnaise (see recipe in this chapter)
2 teaspoons white vinegar
1 teaspoon granulated stevia
½ teaspoon salt
¼ teaspoon ground black pepper
1 (12-ounce) bag dry broccoli slaw
½ cup halved cherry tomatoes

1. In a large mixing bowl, whisk together mayonnaise, vinegar, stevia, salt, and pepper.

2. Add dry slaw and toss to coat.

3. Refrigerate at least 30 minutes before serving.

Smoked Salmon Bites

For some variations on this recipe, use Homemade Mayonnaise in place of the Homemade Ranch Dressing (see recipe in this chapter) or tuna instead of smoked salmon.

INGREDIENTS | SERVES 6 (MAKES 12 BITES)

8 ounces smoked salmon

2 tablespoons Homemade Ranch Dressing (see recipe in this chapter)

¼ cup finely chopped green onions

1 large cucumber, cut into 12 medallions

½ teaspoon ground black pepper

1. Combine salmon, dressing, and green onions in a medium mixing bowl.

2. Top each cucumber slice with salmon mixture. Sprinkle with pepper. Serve immediately.

Where There's Smoke

Smoking is one of the world's oldest preservation techniques. Prior to refrigeration, freezing, and stovetops, people used to expose meats—like salmon—to smoke from wood fires until they were cooked. The smoking process may actually make the fats in salmon more stable, thereby increasing its antioxidant content.

Spiced Nuts

You can make this recipe your own by using any combination of nuts you'd like (with the exception of peanuts).

INGREDIENTS | SERVES 4

½ cup whole almonds
½ cup walnut halves
½ cup whole cashews
1 large egg white
1 teaspoon ground cinnamon
2 tablespoons granulated stevia
½ teaspoon ground nutmeg

Go Nuts

Raw cashews are exceptionally high in copper—¼ cup provides you with 98 percent of the copper you need for the entire day. Copper allows your body to effectively absorb iron and plays a role in the production of melanin, the pigment that gives your skin and hair its color. Copper also helps eliminate free radicals and build connective tissue.

1. Preheat oven to 275°F. Line a baking sheet with parchment paper.

2. Combine nuts in a medium mixing bowl. In a separate bowl, beat egg white. Pour over nuts and toss to coat.

3. In a small bowl, combine cinnamon, stevia, and nutmeg. Sprinkle cinnamon mixture on nuts and toss to combine

4. Lay nuts out in a single layer on baking sheet and bake 25 minutes, stirring occasionally while cooking.

5. Let cool before serving.

Jalapeño Poppers

These aren't your traditional jalapeño poppers, but once you try the combination of jalapeño and creamy avocado, you won't even miss the old version.

INGREDIENTS | SERVES 10

1 large avocado, halved, pitted, and flesh removed

½ teaspoon garlic powder

½ teaspoon onion powder

¼ teaspoon salt

¼ teaspoon ground black pepper

1 teaspoon lemon juice

10 whole large jalapeños, halved and seeded

10 slices turkey bacon

1. Set oven broiler to low.

2. Add avocado, garlic powder, onion powder, salt, pepper, and lemon juice to a medium mixing bowl. Mash with a fork until all ingredients are combined.

3. Scoop 1 teaspoon avocado mixture into each jalapeño half. Cut bacon slices in half.

4. Wrap each half-slice bacon around each jalapeño half and secure with a toothpick. Broil 16 minutes, flipping jalapeños over halfway through cooking.

An Avocado Lesson

Avocados ripen fast, so choose wisely when picking an avocado for this snack. You want one that's deep green and gives slightly to pressure when you press your thumb into it. If the avocado is bright green and rock solid, it's not ready yet. If it's black and mushy, it's too ripe.

Stuffed Tomatoes

Stuffing these cherry tomatoes requires a little bit of patience, but the effort is well worth the payoff.

INGREDIENTS | SERVES 4

20 cherry tomatoes

½ cup chopped fresh basil

1 clove garlic, minced

¼ teaspoon ground black pepper

1 tablespoon olive oil

1. Turn oven broiler to low. Cut tops off cherry tomatoes and scoop out seeds with a small spoon.

2. In a small mixing bowl, mash together basil, garlic, pepper, and oil. Stuff each tomato with basil mixture.

3. Line baking sheet with tomatoes and broil 3–5 minutes or until tomatoes are heated through.

Deviled Eggs

Deviled eggs are a party classic. This recipe gets a clean makeover by swapping out commercial mayonnaise, which contains refined oils and artificial ingredients, with homemade mayonnaise.

INGREDIENTS | SERVES 6

6 hard-boiled large eggs, peeled, halved, and yolks removed

¼ cup Homemade Mayonnaise (see recipe in this chapter)

1 teaspoon white vinegar

1 teaspoon dry mustard

½ teaspoon salt

¼ teaspoon ground black pepper

⅛ teaspoon smoked paprika

1. Put egg yolks in a medium mixing bowl and mash with a fork; then add mayonnaise, vinegar, mustard, salt, and pepper. Continue to mash until combined.

2. Fill each egg white half equally with yolk mixture. Sprinkle with paprika.

The Perfect Hard-Boiled Egg

Hard-boiled eggs are a convenient grab-and-go source of protein, but if you don't cook them right, peeling can be a nightmare. Place eggs in a small saucepan and cover them by 1" with cool water. Allow water to come to a slow boil over medium heat. Once the water has begun to boil, cover, remove from heat, and allow to sit in the hot water for 12 minutes. After 12 minutes, dunk eggs into an ice-water bath and then place under cool water until egg has cooled down completely.

Sugar Snap Peas with Mint

Sugar snap peas are a sweet cross between snow peas and garden peas. They have a crunchy texture with a refreshing taste that is complemented by the mint in this recipe.

INGREDIENTS | SERVES 4

3 teaspoons olive oil

2 cloves garlic, minced

1 pound sugar snap peas

¼ teaspoon salt

¼ teaspoon ground black pepper

3 teaspoons chopped fresh mint

1. Heat olive oil in a medium skillet over medium heat and add garlic. Sauté 3–4 minutes or until fragrant.

2. Add sugar snap peas and continue to sauté until softened, about 4 more minutes.

3. Remove from heat and stir in salt, pepper, and mint. Serve immediately.

Sugar, Sugar Snap Peas

Don't let the "sugar" in sugar snap peas fool you. Sugar snap peas have a very low glycemic index and won't cause a crazy blood sugar rollercoaster. They're also a great source of vitamin K, which helps create healthy new bones and may even reduce your risk of bone fractures.

Dill and Cucumber Salad

Put your own twist on this cucumber salad by adding some of your favorite vegetables— chopped bell peppers and sliced raw zucchini make excellent additions.

INGREDIENTS | SERVES 6

¼ cup Homemade Mayonnaise (see recipe in this chapter)

1 teaspoon granulated stevia

2 teaspoons distilled white vinegar

½ teaspoon ground black pepper

3 tablespoons chopped fresh dill

2 medium cucumbers, thinly sliced

1. Combine all ingredients except cucumbers in a small mixing bowl. Whisk until thoroughly combined.

2. Pour mixture over cucumbers and toss to combine. Refrigerate 30 minutes before serving.

Lemon Pepper Zucchini

This recipe calls for roasting the zucchini, but if you prefer a cold side dish, you can toss all the ingredients together and let it refrigerate for 30 minutes before serving.

INGREDIENTS | SERVES 4

2 small zucchini, thinly sliced

3 tablespoons olive oil

1 tablespoon lemon pepper

1. Preheat oven to 400°F. Line a baking sheet with parchment paper.

2. Toss all ingredients together in a medium mixing bowl. Spread zucchini out in a single layer on baking sheet.

3. Bake 20 minutes or until zucchini is softened but not mushy.

Caramelized Peppers and Onions

This basic Caramelized Peppers and Onions recipe makes a nice addition to any meat entrée, salad, or stir-fry dish.

INGREDIENTS | SERVES

2 tablespoons olive oil

1 medium red bell pepper, seeded and cut into strips

1 medium green bell pepper, seeded and cut into strips

2 medium yellow onions, peeled and cut into strips

¼ teaspoon salt

¼ teaspoon ground black pepper

1. Heat olive oil in a large skillet over medium-high heat. Add sliced peppers and onions and sauté 3–4 minutes or until peppers start to soften. Reduce heat to low and continue cooking.

2. Add salt and pepper and cook 10 more minutes or until peppers and onions completely soften and caramelize.

Roasted Cauliflower

This recipe requires you to roast the entire head of cauliflower whole.

INGREDIENTS | SERVES 6

1 large head cauliflower
3 tablespoons olive oil
½ tablespoon chopped fresh parsley
1 clove garlic, minced
½ teaspoon onion powder
½ teaspoon ground cumin
¼ teaspoon salt
¼ teaspoon ground black pepper

1. Preheat oven to 375°F.

2. Cut off leaves and stem from cauliflower, leaving head intact. Place cauliflower upright in a baking dish.

3. In a small bowl, whisk together remaining ingredients. Brush olive oil mixture over cauliflower, making sure to cover the whole head.

4. Roast until tender, about 60–75 minutes. Allow to cool 5 minutes before serving.

Zucchini Boats

You can make some variations on this recipe by replacing the zucchini with cucumber or even thickly cut slices of red or green bell pepper.

INGREDIENTS | SERVES 6

3 large zucchini
½ cup chopped fresh basil leaves
1 clove garlic, minced
½ cup Homemade Mayonnaise (see recipe in this chapter)
1 tablespoon lemon juice
¼ teaspoon salt
¼ teaspoon ground black pepper
⅛ teaspoon cayenne pepper

1. Preheat oven to 450°F.

2. Cut each zucchini in half lengthwise and then again horizontally. Scoop out seeds with a small spoon.

3. Put remaining ingredients in a medium bowl and stir with a fork until combined. Fill each zucchini boat with mayonnaise mixture.

4. Bake 30 minutes or until zucchini is tender but not mushy.

Water Weight

Zucchini is composed of about 95 percent water, so in addition to filling you up with very few calories, it also serves to hydrate you, helping to get rid of any bloat or excess water weight. Cucumbers are slightly higher in water—consisting of 96 percent.

Sautéed Beet Greens

Beet greens don't often get the love they deserve. Many people buy fresh beets, cut off the tops, and discard the greens, but these leafy greens aren't just nutritious; they're delicious when served up just right.

INGREDIENTS | SERVES 6

3 tablespoons olive oil

2 tablespoons minced shallot

2 cloves garlic, minced

1 pound beet greens, stems removed and chopped

1 tablespoon prepared horseradish

2 teaspoons capers

1 tablespoon fresh lemon juice

¼ teaspoon salt

¼ teaspoon ground black pepper

1. Heat olive oil in a large skillet over medium-high heat. Add shallot and garlic and cook until fragrant, about 3 minutes. Add beet greens and continue to cook until the greens wilt, about 5 minutes.

2. Reduce heat to low and stir in horseradish, capers, lemon juice, salt, and pepper. Continue to cook for 1 minute and serve warm.

The Benefits of Beet Greens

Leafy greens are often lumped into the same nutrition category, but each green has its own nutritional profile and health benefits. Beet greens provide excellent amounts of both calcium and magnesium and are one of the highest plant contributors to iron, providing about 15 percent of your daily needs for the day in 1 cup.

Kale Salad

If you're new to kale, opt for the lacinato variety, which is slightly sweeter and not as bitter as the more popular curly kale.

INGREDIENTS | SERVES 3

2 tablespoons lemon juice

2 teaspoons Dijon mustard

2 cloves garlic, minced

3 canned anchovies, minced

¼ cup olive oil

¼ teaspoon salt

¼ teaspoon ground black pepper

6 cups kale, stems and ribs removed

1. Put all ingredients except kale in a food processor and process until smooth.

2. Pour dressing over kale and massage until kale softens, about 2 minutes. Serve immediately.

Kale for Calcium

Calorie for calorie, kale offers more calcium than milk. Kale is also rich in vitamin A, vitamin K, vitamin C, and fiber. Because of its high fiber content, kale is good for promoting digestion and cleansing the intestines.

Avocado Bites

Bacon and avocado may not sound like a good combination, but don't knock it until you try it. The salty, crispy bacon and smooth, creamy avocado make the perfect pair.

INGREDIENTS | SERVES 4

2 large avocados, halved, pitted, and flesh removed

8 slices turkey bacon, halved

½ teaspoon garlic salt

Precook Your Bacon

If you cook avocado too long, it can turn the avocado bitter. You can shorten the cooking time of this recipe by slightly pre-cooking the bacon—enough that it's partially cooked but still bendable—and then wrapping it around the avocado and putting it in the oven.

1. Preheat oven to 425°F. Line a baking sheet with parchment paper.

2. Cut each avocado into 8 equal-sized slices, making 16 slices total (4 slices per half).

3. Wrap each half-slice bacon around each avocado slice.

4. Place avocado on baking sheet and bake 15 minutes. Turn oven to broil and continue to cook another 2–3 minutes until bacon becomes crispy.

Buffalo Cauliflower Bites

These Buffalo Cauliflower Bites allow you that buffalo wing fix, but with less calories and fat and none of the guilt.

INGREDIENTS | SERVES 6

1 large head cauliflower, cut into florets

1 tablespoon olive oil

½ teaspoon salt

¼ teaspoon ground black pepper

¼ cup hot sauce

1. Preheat oven to 400°F. Line a baking sheet with parchment paper.

2. Combine cauliflower, oil, salt, and pepper on baking sheet and toss to coat. Bake 30 minutes or until cauliflower is fork tender and starting to brown.

3. Remove from oven and toss with hot sauce. Serve immediately.

Spicy Sautéed Kale

Remove the kale ribs and stems before cooking. If you leave them in, this dish can come out tough and hard to chew. The easiest way to free the leaves is to rip them right off the stem and then chop.

INGREDIENTS | SERVES 4

2 tablespoons olive oil

2 cloves garlic, minced

1 large bunch kale, stems removed and leaves roughly chopped

½ cup vegetable broth

½ teaspoon salt

¼ teaspoon ground black pepper

¼ teaspoon red pepper flakes

2 teaspoons cayenne pepper sauce

1. Heat olive oil in a medium saucepan over medium-high heat. Add garlic and sauté until fragrant, about 2 minutes.

2. Add kale to the pan along with the broth. Stir to combine.

3. Cover saucepan and cook 5 minutes. Remove cover and continue cooking until kale is soft and all liquid has evaporated, about 5 more minutes.

4. Add salt, pepper, red pepper flakes, and hot sauce and toss to combine. Serve immediately.

Caramelized Mushrooms

This recipe calls for crimini mushrooms, but you can use any variety of mushroom that you'd like.

INGREDIENTS | SERVES 4

2 tablespoons olive oil

2 cloves garlic, minced

1 pound crimini mushrooms, sliced

1 tablespoon coconut aminos

1. Heat olive oil in a large skillet over medium-high heat. Add garlic and sauté until fragrant, about 3 minutes.

2. Add mushrooms and coconut aminos, stirring to coat evenly. Cook the mushrooms about 4 minutes, allowing them to start to caramelize. Do not stir during this time.

3. Stir once and continue to cook another 5 minutes or until mushrooms reach desired doneness.

Balsamic-Roasted Brussels Sprouts

Brussels sprouts often top the list of most hated vegetables, but it's possible you've just been preparing them all wrong. Try these Balsamic-Roasted Brussels Sprouts, and these mini cabbages may sit atop your most loved vegetables list.

INGREDIENTS | SERVES 4

1 pound Brussels sprouts, cleaned and halved

2 tablespoons olive oil

2 tablespoons balsamic vinegar

½ teaspoon salt

¼ teaspoon freshly ground black pepper

1. Preheat oven to 375°F. Line a baking sheet with parchment paper.

2. Put Brussels sprouts in a large bowl and add remaining ingredients. Toss to combine.

3. Spread out in a single layer on baking sheet and roast 30 minutes or until sprouts are fork tender, turning once while cooking.

Thank the Stink

You may think Brussels sprouts stink—literally—but you can thank that odor for this green vegetable's health benefits. Brussels sprouts contain glucosinolates—cancer-fighting compounds that provide nutritional support for the body's detoxification system. These glucosinolates are also what give Brussels sprouts their distinctive smell.

Fried Cabbage

The variety of cabbage you choose for this recipe isn't as important as making sure to pick one that's fresh. If you go for a napa or Savoy cabbage, make sure the leaves look healthy and have well-defined veins. If you go for a green or red cabbage, choose one whose leaves look tight and compact. Avoid cabbages that look wilted or have browning or slimy leaves.

INGREDIENTS | SERVES 6

6 slices turkey bacon, chopped

1 large white onion, peeled and diced

2 cloves garlic, minced

1 large head cabbage, roughly chopped

1 teaspoon salt

1 teaspoon ground black pepper

¼ teaspoon red pepper flakes (optional)

Moon Power!

Ancient healers claimed that the health benefits of cabbage came from the power of the moon, since this vegetable grew in the moonlight. It may actually be the high content of vitamin K, vitamin C, and sulfur that are responsible for cabbage's notable health benefits, but either way, you should be eating more of it.

1. Heat a medium skillet over medium-high heat. Add bacon and cook until crispy. Add onion and garlic and cook until onion starts to caramelize, about 7 minutes.

2. Add cabbage and continue to cook until cabbage softens, about 5 minutes. Sprinkle on spices and stir to incorporate.

3. Serve immediately.

Homemade Mayonnaise

You can use olive oil in this recipe in place of avocado oil. If you prefer a milder taste, opt for extra-light olive oil. If you like mayonnaise with a strong olive oil flavor, go for extra-virgin olive oil.

**INGREDIENTS | MAKES 1¼ CUPS
(SERVES 10)**

1 large egg, room temperature

Juice from ½ large lemon, room temperature

½ teaspoon dry mustard

½ teaspoon salt

¼ teaspoon ground black pepper

1 cup avocado oil

Creating an Emulsion

Mayonnaise is made by creating an emulsion—a mixture of oil and water (from the eggs). Allowing the eggs and lemon juice to reach room temperature before preparing this recipe will make it easier for the oil and water to mix, which isn't a simple feat. If the ingredients are cold, the emulsion may fail and you'll be left with a runny mess.

1. Combine egg and lemon juice in a narrow container and let sit 30 minutes.

2. Add dry mustard, salt, pepper, and avocado oil. Insert an immersion blender into mixture until it hits the bottom of the container.

3. Turn on blender and blend 30 seconds. As the mixture starts to emulsify, pull the blender out of the mixture slightly to mix in the oil on the top.

4. Transfer to a tightly sealed container and store in the refrigerator for up to 7 days.

CHAPTER 11

MD Stage 3 Breakfast

Coconut Oatmeal

Steel-cut oats require a longer cooking time than old-fashioned oats, but it's worth the wait. Steel-cut oats have a lower glycemic index, so they won't affect your blood sugar as significantly as old-fashioned oats do.

INGREDIENTS | SERVES 4

1 cup steel-cut oats

1½ cups water

1½ cups coconut milk

1 teaspoon vanilla extract

1 teaspoon granulated stevia

½ cup unsweetened toasted coconut flakes

2 tablespoons crushed walnuts

1. Combine oats, water, and coconut milk in a medium saucepan and heat over medium-high heat, stirring frequently until mixture comes to a boil.

2. Reduce heat to low and simmer 20 minutes or until oats are soft.

3. Remove from heat and stir in vanilla and stevia.

4. Divide into serving bowls and sprinkle with toasted coconut and walnuts.

Almond Butter, Coconut, and Raspberry Roll-Ups

This combination may sound a little "out there," but give it a try. You're likely to be pleasantly surprised.

INGREDIENTS | SERVES 2

2 sprouted-grain tortillas

2 tablespoons almond butter (no sugar added)

1 cup fresh raspberries

½ cup shaved unsweetened coconut

1. Warm tortillas in the microwave 20 seconds. Remove from microwave and spread each tortilla with 1 tablespoon almond butter.

2. Top each tortilla with ½ cup raspberries and ¼ cup shaved coconut. Roll up and secure with a toothpick.

3. Serve immediately.

MCTs—The Superfat?

Coconut was once deemed "unhealthy" because of its high content of saturated fat. It's now known that most of that saturated fat is in a unique form called medium-chain triglycerides (MCTs). Medium-chain triglycerides are easy to digest, and your body prefers to use them right up as energy instead of storing them as fat. A study in the *American Journal of Clinical Nutrition* reported that eating MCTs from coconut products can actually increase your metabolism three times as much as eating the long-chain triglycerides found in vegetable oils. MCTs can also help the body burn off excess fat.

Vegetable-Packed Scrambled Eggs

Having scrambled eggs packed with vegetables is a great way to get in plenty of vegetables first thing in the morning. The combination of protein and vegetables starts your day off right!

INGREDIENTS | SERVES 2

1 tablespoon coconut oil
½ medium zucchini, diced
½ cup chopped yellow onion
½ cup chopped mushrooms
½ cup diced red bell peppers
1 cup chopped spinach
½ cup chopped tomatoes
4 large eggs
½ teaspoon salt
¼ teaspoon ground black pepper

1. Heat coconut oil in a medium skillet over medium-high heat. Add zucchini, onion, mushrooms, and bell peppers and sauté until soft, about 5 minutes.

2. Add spinach and tomatoes and cook until spinach is wilted, about 3 minutes.

3. While vegetables are cooking, whisk eggs in a small bowl with salt and pepper. Pour eggs over vegetables and scramble until eggs are cooked through. Serve immediately.

Veg Out

Studies show that when you eat vegetables with breakfast, you're more likely to meet your micronutrient needs for the entire day and make better choices for the rest of the day.

Coconut Flour Pancakes with Berry Compote

Coconut flour is highly absorbable, so you only need a small amount in these coconut flour pancakes. Once topped with the berry compote, you won't even need maple syrup.

INGREDIENTS | SERVES 2

¼ cup coconut flour

¼ teaspoon baking soda

⅛ teaspoon salt

½ teaspoon ground cinnamon

½ teaspoon apple cider vinegar

⅓ cup coconut milk

3 large eggs

2 tablespoons coconut oil, melted, divided

½ teaspoon vanilla extract

½ cup frozen mixed berries

1 teaspoon granulated stevia

1. Mix dry ingredients—coconut flour, baking soda, salt, and cinnamon—in a small bowl.

2. In a medium bowl, whisk together vinegar, coconut milk, eggs, 1 tablespoon coconut oil, and vanilla. Set aside.

3. Heat a small saucepan over medium heat. Add in frozen berries. Use a spatula to crush berries as they begin to heat up. Add stevia and continue smashing with spatula until berries reach desired consistency. Set aside.

4. Heat up a medium skillet over medium heat and add remaining coconut oil. Combine wet and dry pancake ingredients.

5. Drop batter by ⅛ cupfuls onto hot skillet. Cook 3–4 minutes and then flip over and cook another 3–4 minutes or until pancake is browned and cooked through.

6. Top pancakes with berry compote. Serve immediately.

Cacao Power Smoothie

Turn this smoothie into an even bigger energy booster by adding a teaspoon of spirulina into the mix before blending.

INGREDIENTS | SERVES 2

1 cup almond milk

1½ cups spinach

¾ cup frozen berry mixture (blackberries, blueberries, raspberries, and cherries)

1 tablespoon ground flaxseed

1 teaspoon chia seeds

2 teaspoons raw cacao powder

Combine all ingredients in blender and blend until smooth. Serve immediately.

Fruit Salad with Coconut Cream

Don't forget to chill the coconut milk! If you use coconut milk that's at room temperature, it won't whip up as easily and may not form peaks at all.

INGREDIENTS | SERVES 2

¼ cup blueberries

¼ cup blackberries

¼ cup raspberries

1 tablespoon fresh lemon juice

½ cup chilled full-fat coconut milk

1 teaspoon granulated stevia

½ teaspoon vanilla extract

1. Combine blueberries, blackberries, and raspberries in a medium bowl. Pour lemon juice on top and toss to combine.

2. Put coconut milk in a separate chilled bowl. Beat with a handheld beater until peaks begin to form, about 3 minutes. Beat in stevia and vanilla extract just until combined. Do not overbeat.

3. Divide berries evenly between two serving bowls and top each with half the coconut cream. Serve immediately.

Peach Avocado Smoothie

Don't let the avocado turn you off from trying this smoothie. It provides essential fats while giving the smoothie a nice, creamy texture—and you can't even taste it.

INGREDIENTS | SERVES 2

½ cup frozen peaches

1 cup coconut water

½ medium avocado, pitted and flesh removed

½ cup almond milk

1 cup baby spinach

Combine all ingredients in a blender and blend until smooth. Serve immediately.

Homemade Almond Milk

Like commercial boxed coconut milks, the prepared almond milk sold in stores is often full of less than ideal additives. The solution? Make your own! Simply soak 1 cup raw almonds in water for at least 12 hours. Add soaked almonds to a blender along with 3½ cups filtered water and 1 teaspoon vanilla extract and blend for 1 minute. Strain milk through a nut milk bag or cheesecloth and you're done.

Sweet Potato Hash with Fried Eggs and Avocado

Sweet potatoes, eggs, and avocado are the perfect breakfast trifecta. They provide a balance of starchy carbohydrates, protein, and healthy fats that will keep you full and satisfied.

INGREDIENTS | SERVES 2

1 large sweet potato, peeled
½ teaspoon garlic powder
½ teaspoon onion powder
½ teaspoon coarse sea salt
2 tablespoons coconut oil, divided
4 large eggs
½ medium avocado, pitted, flesh removed, and sliced thinly

1. Grate sweet potato with a cheese grater or with the grating attachment on a food processor. Mix shredded sweet potato with garlic powder, onion powder, and sea salt in a medium bowl. Toss to combine.

2. Heat 1 tablespoon coconut oil in a medium skillet over medium-high heat. Once oil is hot, add sweet potato. Sauté until tender, about 12 minutes, stirring occasionally. Remove potatoes from skillet with a slotted spoon and divide between two serving plates.

3. Melt remaining 1 tablespoon coconut oil in the same skillet. Crack eggs into skillet once oil is hot. Cook 2 minutes and then flip over and cook another 2 minutes, using care not to break the yolks. Put 2 eggs on each plate over the sweet potatoes.

4. Divide the avocado evenly over each egg. Serve immediately.

Stuffed Omelet

Make this omelet your go-to breakfast by substituting any of the listed vegetables with your favorites.

INGREDIENTS | SERVES 2

1 tablespoon olive oil

¼ cup chopped white onion

½ medium red bell pepper, seeded and diced

½ medium green bell pepper, seeded and diced

1 cup broccoli florets

1 cup chopped spinach

½ cup chopped white mushrooms

4 large eggs

½ teaspoon salt

¼ teaspoon ground black pepper

1. Heat olive oil in a medium skillet over medium heat. Add onion, peppers, and broccoli. Cover skillet and allow to steam 2 minutes. Remove cover and sauté until all vegetables are tender, about 5 more minutes.

2. Add spinach and mushrooms and sauté until mushrooms are tender and spinach is wilted, about 4 minutes. Remove vegetables from skillet with slotted spoon.

3. In a small bowl, whisk together eggs, salt, and pepper. Pour in skillet and allow to cook, tilting the skillet to allow uncooked egg in the middle to fall to the sides. Flip eggs over and cook another 2–3 minutes or until fully cooked through. Place vegetables on one side of cooked egg and flip the other side over to cover them.

4. Remove from heat and serve immediately.

Nutty Oats

The combination of protein, fiber, and healthy fat in this breakfast will help fill you up while also satisfying that craving for some morning comfort food.

INGREDIENTS | SERVES 2

1 cup steel-cut oats

1 cup almond milk

1 cup water

½ cup blueberries

1 teaspoon ground cinnamon

½ teaspoon ground allspice

½ teaspoon vanilla extract

1 tablespoon chopped walnuts

1 tablespoon chopped almonds

Combine all ingredients in a slow cooker and cook on low 8 hours.

The Unique Walnut

The form of vitamin E found in walnuts is somewhat unique. Most vitamin E–rich foods contain alpha-tocopherol, while walnuts are rich in gamma-tocopherol. While both forms of vitamin E are considered heart-healthy, gamma-tocopherol has been shown to be particularly effective in reducing the risk of heart problems.

Chocolate-Covered Blueberry Smoothie

This smoothie will make you think you're eating chocolate-covered blueberries in liquid form. Switch up the flavor profile by using any combination of berries.

INGREDIENTS | SERVES 2

1 cup frozen blueberries

1½ cups unsweetened chocolate almond milk

1 tablespoon raw cacao powder

½ teaspoon vanilla extract

Combine all ingredients in a blender and blend until smooth. Serve immediately.

Good Things Come in Small Packages

Blueberries are one of the most nutrient-dense, antioxidant-rich foods in the world. One of the most notable nutritional components of blueberries is gallic acid, a powerful antiviral and antifungal compound that also acts as an antioxidant. In addition to other nutritional benefits, gallic acid is considered neuroprotective, which means that it can protect your brain from degeneration, oxidative stress, and neurotoxicity.

Root Vegetable Frittata

Root vegetables are one of the most underappreciated foods around. These vegetables are not only nutritional powerhouses, but they're also inexpensive and available in the winter when it can be difficult to find other fresh vegetables.

INGREDIENTS | SERVES 4

¼ cup chopped shallots
1 clove garlic, minced
½ cup diced carrots
½ cup diced sweet potatoes
½ cup diced turnips
2 tablespoons olive oil
½ teaspoon salt
½ teaspoon ground black pepper
½ teaspoon ground cinnamon
8 large eggs
2 tablespoons chopped fresh parsley

1. Preheat oven to 375°F.

2. Combine shallots, garlic, carrots, sweet potatoes, turnips, olive oil, salt, pepper, and cinnamon in an 8" × 8" baking dish. Toss to combine.

3. Bake in oven 40 minutes or until vegetables are fork tender. Remove from oven.

4. Beat eggs and parsley together in a medium bowl and pour over cooked vegetables, making sure eggs spread evenly. Return to oven and bake 15 minutes or until egg sets. Allow to cool 5 minutes before serving.

Overnight Berry Oatmeal

This recipe doesn't require any cooking—you just prepare everything the night before and then you'll have a healthy breakfast ready for you in the morning. You can enjoy this recipe cold, but if you'd prefer to heat it up, just put it in a saucepan with a little coconut or almond milk and stir until warmed through.

INGREDIENTS | SERVES 1

¾ cup coconut or almond milk

½ cup old-fashioned oats

1 teaspoon chia seeds

⅛ teaspoon salt

⅛ teaspoon ground cinnamon

⅛ teaspoon vanilla extract

⅓ cup fresh blueberries

1 tablespoon slivered almonds

1. Combine milk, oats, chia seeds, salt, cinnamon, vanilla, and blueberries in a Mason jar or another container with a lid. Tighten the lid and shake so that everything is combined.

2. Put in the refrigerator and let sit at least 6 hours or overnight.

3. In the morning, top with slivered almonds.

Time-Saving Trick

Prepare a week's worth of breakfast in advance by filling up seven different Mason jars with this oatmeal mixture, without the milk. Store each jar tightly sealed in the pantry and then add milk and shake it up the night before you're ready to eat it and store it in the fridge.

Pumpkin Waffles

You can use freshly cooked mashed pumpkin or canned pumpkin purée. If you're using canned pumpkin purée, make sure you're getting pure pumpkin and not pumpkin pie filling, which often contains added sweeteners.

INGREDIENTS | SERVES 2

3 large eggs
1 cup mashed pumpkin
½ cup cashew butter (no sugar added)
1 tablespoon coconut flour
1 teaspoon vanilla extract
1 teaspoon pumpkin pie spice
½ teaspoon baking soda
2 teaspoons coconut oil
1 cup mixed berries (optional)

1. Preheat waffle maker.

2. Separate egg yolks and whites reserving each in separate bowls.

3. In a large mixing bowl, mix together egg yolks, mashed pumpkin, cashew butter, coconut flour, vanilla, pumpkin pie spice, and baking soda. Blend with a handheld mixer 2 minutes.

4. In a separate bowl, beat the egg whites with an electric mixer until peaks form, about 3 minutes. Fold egg whites into pumpkin mixture until combined.

5. Grease waffle maker with coconut oil and pour ½ waffle batter on top. Cook until browned and waffle comes off of maker easily, about 6 minutes. Repeat with the remaining batter.

6. Serve with fresh berries on top if desired.

Spirulina Avocado Smoothie

Many grocery stores have frozen, pitted cherries available in the freezer section. If you can't find frozen cherries, get some fresh cherries, but make sure to remove the pits before blending.

INGREDIENTS | SERVES 2

1 cup coconut water

½ medium avocado, pitted and flesh removed

2 teaspoons spirulina

½ cup blueberries

½ cup pitted cherries

1 teaspoon raw cacao

Combine all ingredients in a blender and blend until smooth. Serve immediately.

Cherry Picker

The anthocyanins in cherries help reduce insulin resistance and increase glucose tolerance while also fighting widespread inflammation by inhibiting the enzymes that cause it.

Nut Cereal with Coconut Milk and Berries

This grain-free cereal is so much more satisfying than the refined carbohydrate-laden stuff that you may be used to.

INGREDIENTS | SERVES 6

1 cup cashews

½ cup almonds

¼ cup sunflower seeds

¼ cup pumpkin seeds

½ cup unsweetened coconut flakes

2 tablespoons coconut oil, melted

1 teaspoon vanilla extract

½ teaspoon salt

¾ teaspoon ground cinnamon

3 cups coconut milk

3 cups blueberries

Save Those Pumpkin Seeds!

It's estimated that up to 80 percent of Americans are deficient in magnesium—a mineral that's involved in energy production, protein synthesis, relaxation, proper bowel function, and cell signaling in your body. Just ¼ cup of pumpkin seeds contains almost half of the magnesium you need for the entire day.

1. Preheat oven to 300°F. Line a baking sheet with parchment paper.

2. Combine cashews, almonds, sunflower seeds, and pumpkin seeds in a food processor and pulse a few times to break the nuts down into smaller pieces. Remove from food processor and toss in a medium bowl with coconut flakes, coconut oil, vanilla extract, salt, and cinnamon.

3. Spread mixture out on baking sheet. Cook 35 minutes, flipping once, until mixture starts to brown. Remove from oven and allow to cool.

4. For each serving, put ½ cup nut mixture in a bowl; cover with ½ cup coconut milk and ½ cup fresh berries.

Mixed-Berry Smoothie

Try some variations on this basic antioxidant-rich smoothie by replacing almond butter with cashew butter or sunflower seed butter and adding a couple of teaspoons of raw cacao powder.

INGREDIENTS | SERVES 2

¼ cup pitted cherries

¼ cup blueberries

¼ cup blackberries

¼ cup raspberries

1 cup coconut water

¼ cup coconut milk

1 cup baby kale

1 teaspoon fresh lemon juice

2 teaspoons almond butter (no sugar added)

Put all ingredients in a blender and blend until smooth. Serve immediately.

Monkey Salad

Traditional monkey salad uses sliced bananas as a base, and that's where the "monkey" name comes from. Because bananas are high in carbohydrates, this version leaves them out; the flavor is so good, you won't miss them.

INGREDIENTS | SERVES 4

2 tablespoons coconut oil

½ cup unsweetened coconut flakes

½ cup raw unsalted cashews

½ cup raw unsalted almonds

¼ cup almond butter, melted

1. Melt coconut oil in a medium skillet over medium heat. Add coconut flakes and sauté until lightly browned, 3–4 minutes.

2. Add cashews and almonds and sauté 2 minutes. Remove from heat and drizzle with melted almond butter. Serve immediately.

Sweet Treat

Monkey Salad is the perfect sweet and satisfying treat. It's loaded with healthy fats that help keep you full between meals, and it's so easy to take on the go.

Old-Fashioned Peach Coconut Oatmeal

If you want to sweeten this breakfast up a bit, you can add some vanilla extract, cinnamon, and a few drops of liquid stevia extract.

INGREDIENTS | SERVES 1

1 cup coconut milk
⅔ cup old-fashioned oats
2 tablespoons unsweetened coconut flakes
1 tablespoon chopped walnuts
½ cup chopped peaches

1. Pour coconut milk into a small saucepan and bring to a boil over high heat. Once milk starts boiling, add oats, coconut flakes, and walnuts. Allow mixture to come back to a boil, then reduce heat to medium and cook 5 minutes.

2. Stir in peaches, cook 1 more minute, and then remove from heat. Serve immediately.

Sprouted French Toast with Coconut Whipped Cream

This cleaned-up version of French toast will prevent you from feeling deprived of a hearty Sunday breakfast.

INGREDIENTS | SERVES 2

½ cup chilled full-fat canned coconut milk
1 teaspoon granulated stevia
2½ teaspoons vanilla extract, divided
2 large eggs
½ teaspoon ground cinnamon
2 slices sprouted-grain bread
1 tablespoon chopped pecans

Nutrient-Packed Pecans

Pecans are loaded with nutrients. They contain more than nineteen different vitamins and minerals, including vitamin A, vitamin E, B vitamins, calcium, magnesium, phosphorus, and zinc. Just a handful of pecans a day can help lower cholesterol numbers.

1. Put chilled coconut milk, stevia, and ½ teaspoon vanilla in a chilled medium bowl. Beat with a handheld beater until peaks begin to form, about 3 minutes.

2. Whisk eggs, remaining 2 teaspoons vanilla, and cinnamon together in a small bowl. Soak each sprouted-bread slice in the mixture, making sure to coat both sides.

3. Transfer bread to a medium skillet and cook over medium heat, flipping once so that both sides are browned, about 3 minutes on each side.

4. Transfer French toast to a plate and top each slice with half the coconut whipped cream and ½ tablespoon pecans. Serve warm.

Berry Chia Pudding

A single ounce of chia seeds contains 11 grams of fiber—almost half your needs for the entire day. The tiny seeds are also loaded with protein and omega-3 fatty acids as well as a combination of vitamins and minerals.

INGREDIENTS | SERVES 4

1 cup full-fat coconut milk

1 cup almond milk

1 teaspoon vanilla extract

1 tablespoon unsweetened cocoa powder

1 teaspoon granulated stevia

2 tablespoons unsweetened coconut flakes

½ cup chia seeds

¼ cup fresh berries

1. Combine coconut milk, almond milk, vanilla, cocoa powder, and stevia in blender and blend.

2. Add coconut flakes and chia seeds to mixture and stir until evenly dispersed. Cover and refrigerate 8 hours. Top with fresh berries immediately before serving.

Coconut Chia Smoothie

You can turn this into a chocolate coconut chia smoothie by adding a couple teaspoons of unsweetened cocoa powder before blending.

INGREDIENTS | SERVES 1

1 cup full-fat canned coconut milk

2 tablespoons chia seeds

2 tablespoons coconut water

¼ cup frozen blueberries

Place all ingredients in a blender and blend until smooth.

Nut Butter Berries

This recipe may seem out of the ordinary, but cashew butter and berries make quite the pleasant pair. It's like peanut butter and jelly in a bowl, but with better ingredients.

INGREDIENTS | SERVES 2

4 tablespoons unsweetened cashew butter

2 cups mixed fresh berries

2 tablespoons toasted coconut flakes

2 teaspoons cacao nibs

1. Melt cashew butter in a microwave-safe bowl 30–60 seconds or until thinned.

2. Add berries and toss to coat.

3. Sprinkle coconut flakes and cacao nibs on top. Serve warm.

Berries for Brain Power

According to research published in the medical journal *Annals of Neurology*, women who ate one serving of blueberries or two servings of strawberries per week experienced less mental decline than women who skipped the berries. The compounds in berries credited for the benefit—called anthocyanidins—are able to cross the blood-brain barrier and reach the memory and learning centers in the brain.

Breakfast Egg Salad

There's no doubt you've heard of the classic lunch favorite—the BLT. This breakfast recipe is a spin on that, but without the bread and with nutrient-dense avocado instead.

INGREDIENTS | SERVES 2

1 large avocado, pitted, flesh removed, and diced

2 hard-boiled large eggs, peeled and chopped

4 slices cooked turkey bacon, crumbled

1 medium tomato, seeded and diced

2 teaspoons Homemade Mayonnaise (see recipe in Chapter 10)

¼ teaspoon salt

¼ teaspoon ground black pepper

Combine all ingredients together in a medium bowl and toss to combine, using care not to mash the avocado.

Ham and Egg Breakfast Sandwich

This simple breakfast sandwich is packed with protein and easy to make on a busy day when you're crunched for time.

INGREDIENTS | SERVES 1

1 teaspoon olive oil

1 tablespoon minced yellow onion

2 large eggs, lightly beaten

2 (approximately 2 ounces) slices deli ham (sugar-free)

½ cup chopped spinach

2 teaspoons yellow mustard

Make It Simple

Research shows that people are more likely to eat breakfast if easy-to-prepare breakfast items are available in the house. People who eat breakfast are also less likely to snack during the day. This breakfast sandwich only takes minutes, so you'll be able to start your day on the right track.

1. Heat olive oil in a medium skillet over medium heat. Add onion and sauté until translucent, about 4 minutes. Add eggs and scramble until completely cooked through, about 4 more minutes. Remove from heat.

2. Lay ham slices flat on a plate and scoop half the eggs on each slice. Top with half the spinach and mustard and roll. Secure with a toothpick.

CHAPTER 12

MD Stage 3 Lunch

Almond-Crusted Cod

After you try this Almond-Crusted Cod, you'll never go back to breading with regular bread crumbs.

INGREDIENTS | SERVES 2

2 large egg whites
¼ teaspoon garlic powder
¼ teaspoon lemon pepper
¼ teaspoon dried parsley
⅛ teaspoon salt
⅛ teaspoon ground black pepper
¼ cup ground raw almonds
2 (6-ounce) cod fillets
2 tablespoons olive oil
½ large lemon
2 sprigs parsley (optional)

1. Beat the egg whites in a small shallow bowl and set aside.

2. Combine garlic powder, lemon pepper, parsley, salt, pepper, and almonds in a separate shallow bowl.

3. Dip each fillet in egg white and then coat with almond mixture on both sides.

4. Heat olive oil in a medium skillet over medium heat. Add coated fillets and cook 3–4 minutes on each side or until cod is golden and flakes easily.

5. Remove from heat and transfer to serving dish. Squeeze fresh lemon juice on each fillet and top with sprigs of parsley if desired.

Chicken Fajitas

You can also make these Chicken Fajitas appropriate for Stage 2 by replacing the sprouted-grain tortillas with lettuce wraps.

INGREDIENTS | SERVES 2

1 teaspoon ground cumin

½ teaspoon salt

1 teaspoon garlic powder

1 teaspoon onion powder

½ teaspoon red pepper flakes

3 tablespoons olive oil, divided

2 tablespoons fresh lime juice

8 ounces boneless skinless chicken breasts, cut into 2" strips

½ medium red bell pepper, seeded and julienned

½ medium green bell pepper, seeded and julienned

1 small yellow onion, peeled and julienned

1½ tablespoons coconut aminos

4 (6") sprouted-grain tortillas

⅓ cup chopped cilantro

½ medium avocado, pitted, flesh removed, and sliced thinly

1. Combine cumin, salt, garlic powder, onion powder, and red pepper flakes in a gallon-sized plastic bag and shake to mix thoroughly.

2. Add 1½ tablespoons olive oil, lime juice, and chicken and shake to coat. Place in refrigerator at least 1 hour (up to 24 hours).

3. Heat remaining olive oil in a large skillet over medium heat. Add bell peppers and onion and sauté until soft, about 5 minutes.

4. Add chicken to pepper and onion mixture and cook until chicken is no longer pink, about 7 minutes.

5. Add coconut aminos to pan and allow to cook down, about 3 more minutes. Remove mixture from heat.

6. Prepare fajitas by topping each tortilla with chicken and pepper mixture, cilantro, and avocado. Serve immediately.

Don't Skip the Cilantro!

In addition to being a powerful cleansing agent, cilantro has been shown to improve sleep quality, reduce anxiety, help lower blood sugar, and decrease widespread oxidative stress on the body.

Cobb Salad

If you prefer, you can pair this Cobb Salad with the Homemade Ranch Dressing found in Chapter 10.

INGREDIENTS | SERVES 2

4 cups chopped romaine lettuce

½ cup grape tomatoes, cut in half

½ cup chopped red onion

2 slices cooked nitrate-free turkey bacon, chopped

2 hard-boiled large eggs, peeled and chopped

½ medium avocado, pitted, flesh removed, and sliced thinly

2 teaspoons olive oil

Juice from ½ large lemon

⅛ teaspoon salt

⅛ teaspoon ground black pepper

1. Combine lettuce, tomatoes, onion, bacon, eggs, and avocado in a large bowl. Toss until all ingredients are incorporated.

2. In a small bowl, whisk together, olive oil, lemon juice, salt, and pepper. Add to lettuce mixture and toss to combine.

3. Divide into two separate bowls. Serve immediately.

Salmon and Spinach Salad with Pumpkin Seeds

Canned salmon is an easy, convenient way to get in your omega-3 fatty acids. Keep a can in your drawer at work or even in the car for a quick boost of nutrition on the go.

INGREDIENTS | SERVES 2

2 teaspoons olive oil

Juice from ½ large lemon

½ teaspoon dried oregano

½ teaspoon dried basil

4 cups baby spinach

½ cup pumpkin seeds, raw and unsalted

1 (6-ounce) can pink salmon

1. In a small bowl, whisk together olive oil, lemon juice, oregano, and basil.

2. Place spinach in a large bowl. Pour the dressing over it and massage until spinach starts to wilt, about 3 minutes.

3. Add pumpkin seeds and salmon. Toss until combined.

Choosing a Canned Salmon

Just like with fresh salmon, it's best to choose a canned salmon that is wild-caught instead of farm-raised. Choosing a canned salmon that contains the bones will increase the calcium content of your meal, and they're so small you won't even notice them.

Beef and Broccoli Stir-Fry

*This stir-fry has all the flavor of the traditional beef and broccoli
dish, but without any additives, soy, or MSG.*

INGREDIENTS | SERVES 4

⅓ cup fish sauce

2 teaspoons toasted sesame oil

4 teaspoons coconut aminos, divided

3 cloves garlic, minced and divided

1 pound boneless round steak, cut into thin 2" strips

2 teaspoons coconut oil

1 small yellow onion, peeled and chopped

4 cups fresh broccoli florets

1 teaspoon ground ginger

1 teaspoon toasted sesame seeds

Ginger: The Stomach Soother

Ginger is known as a stomach remedy because it's been used for centuries to treat all sorts of stomach problems, including upset stomach, motion sickness, morning sickness, nausea, gas, diarrhea, colic, and loss of appetite.

1. In a large bowl, mix together fish sauce, sesame oil, 2 teaspoons coconut aminos, and half the garlic. Add steak to bowl, making sure all meat is covered, and marinate in the refrigerator 1 hour.

2. Heat coconut oil in a large skillet or wok over medium-high heat. Add onion and sauté until soft, about 4 minutes. Add broccoli and sauté until broccoli is soft but still crisp, about 5 more minutes.

3. Remove beef from marinade and add to broccoli and onion mixture, along with remaining coconut aminos, remaining garlic, and ginger. Stir well and sauté until beef is cooked, about 7 minutes. Remove from heat and sprinkle with toasted sesame seeds.

4. Serve immediately.

Thai Coconut Spaghetti Squash

This twist on a traditional pad Thai uses sunflower seeds in place of peanuts and spaghetti squash in place of rice noodles.

INGREDIENTS | SERVES 6

1 medium spaghetti squash (about 3 pounds), cut in half lengthwise

¾ cup chicken broth

¾ cup full-fat canned coconut milk

2 tablespoons fish sauce

1 tablespoon coconut aminos

1 tablespoon white vinegar

3 tablespoons creamy sunflower seed butter (no sugar added)

1 teaspoon minced fresh ginger

1 teaspoon toasted sesame oil

Juice from 1 small lime

½ teaspoon ground black pepper

1 tablespoon arrowroot powder

1 tablespoon light olive oil

1 clove garlic, minced

2 cups matchstick carrots

2 cups bean sprouts

1 bunch chopped scallions, green parts only

½ cup chopped, raw, and unsalted sunflower seeds

Sunflower Seeds Aren't Just for the Baseball Field

Sunflower seeds are an excellent source of selenium, a mineral that's known to effectively combat several different types of cancer. They also contain magnesium, copper, and calcium—three minerals that work in conjunction to keep your bones strong.

1. Preheat oven to 400°F.

2. Place squash cut-side up on a baking sheet. Bake until squash is tender, about 30–45 minutes depending on the size of the squash. Peel squash away from skin with a fork and reserve strands in a bowl.

3. While squash is cooking, combine broth, coconut milk, fish sauce, coconut aminos, vinegar, sunflower seed butter, ginger, sesame oil, lime juice, and pepper in a medium saucepan over medium-high heat. Allow to come to a boil. Whisk in arrowroot and continue boiling until sauce thickens, about 5 minutes, stirring constantly. Once sauce thickens, reduce heat to low and allow to simmer.

4. Heat olive oil in a medium skillet over medium-high heat. Add garlic and sauté until fragrant, about 3 minutes. Add carrots and continue to sauté until carrots become tender, about 4 minutes. Add sprouts, scallions, and spaghetti squash strands. Toss until combined.

5. Add sauce and sunflower seeds to spaghetti squash mixture and stir over low heat until sauce is incorporated and all ingredients are warmed through, about 5 minutes. Serve immediately.

Quinoa-Stuffed Peppers

If you use vegetable broth in favor of chicken broth for this
recipe, it's entirely vegan and vegetarian-friendly.

INGREDIENTS | SERVES 4

½ cup quinoa, rinsed and drained

1 cup chicken or vegetable broth

1 tablespoon olive oil

1 small yellow onion, peeled and minced

2 cloves garlic, minced

1 medium zucchini, diced

1 (15-ounce) can black beans, drained
and rinsed

½ teaspoon red pepper flakes

10 cherry tomatoes, chopped

1 cup tomato sauce (no sugar added)

½ teaspoon salt

¼ teaspoon ground black pepper

4 medium bell peppers (green or red),
tops cut off and seeded

1. Preheat oven to 350°F. Line a baking dish with parchment paper.

2. Combine quinoa and broth in a medium saucepan and bring to a boil over high heat. Once mixture starts boiling, cover and reduce heat to low. Allow to simmer 15–20 minutes or until all broth is absorbed and quinoa is soft and fluffy.

3. Heat olive oil in a medium skillet over medium heat. Add onion, garlic, and zucchini and sauté until softened, about 5 minutes. Add remaining ingredients and stir to combine. Continue cooking over medium-low heat, allowing mixture to simmer 10 minutes.

4. Remove vegetable mixture from heat and stir in quinoa. Mix until combined. Place each pepper upright in baking dish and fill with equal amounts quinoa mixture.

5. Cover baking dish with foil and bake 20 minutes or until peppers are tender and filling is bubbling. Serve immediately.

Hummus and Vegetable Sprouted Wrap

This is another vegan and vegetarian-friendly recipe that you could also make appeal to the meat lover by adding some sliced roasted turkey or roast beef.

INGREDIENTS | SERVES 2

6 tablespoons prepared hummus (no sugar added)

2 sprouted-grain tortillas

1 cup pea shoots

½ cup matchstick carrots

10 cherry tomatoes, cut in half

¼ cup sliced black olives

½ medium avocado, pitted, flesh removed, and sliced thinly

¼ cup sliced roasted red peppers

1. Spread 3 tablespoons hummus on each tortilla. Top each tortilla with ½ cup pea shoots, ¼ cup carrots, 5 cherry tomatoes, ⅛ cup olives, ¼ avocado, and ⅛ cup red pepper.

2. Roll tortilla into a wrap and secure with a toothpick. Serve immediately.

Mighty Little Sprouts

Sprouts, like pea shoots, are often nicknamed "nature's perfect food" because of their extremely dense nutritional profile. At this early stage of life, sprouts, which are the beginning of the flower or vegetable they'll eventually become, are full of energy and the vitamins and minerals they need to grow. Pea shoots in particular are rich in protease inhibitors—compounds that can inhibit substances that promote cancer.

Chicken, White Bean, and Lime Salad

The flavors in this recipe develop even more the longer they sit. If you have some extra time, let this recipe sit overnight before you eat it.

INGREDIENTS | SERVES 2

1 (12.5-ounce) can chicken breast

1 cup cannellini beans, drained and rinsed

Juice from 1 medium lime

½ teaspoon seasoned salt

¼ teaspoon ground black pepper

3 tablespoons Homemade Mayonnaise (see recipe in Chapter 10)

1 stalk celery, finely diced

1 tablespoon chopped parsley

Mix all ingredients in a bowl and stir until combined. Chill 30 minutes before serving.

Root Vegetable Quinoa

You can up the protein and fiber content of this vegetarian dish by adding some cooked beans or chickpeas.

INGREDIENTS | SERVES 4

1 small sweet potato, peeled and diced

1 medium beet, peeled and diced

½ cup diced butternut squash

½ cup diced parsnips

1 tablespoon olive oil

½ teaspoon ground cinnamon

1 cup quinoa, rinsed and drained

2 cups vegetable broth

1 tablespoon chopped parsley

1. Preheat oven to 400°F. Line baking sheet with foil.

2. Combine vegetables in a large bowl and toss with olive oil and cinnamon. Spread in a single layer on baking sheet and bake 20–25 minutes or until vegetables are tender.

3. While vegetables are cooking, combine quinoa and broth in a medium saucepan over medium-high heat. Bring to a boil, then reduce heat to low, cover, and allow to simmer 20 minutes or until water is absorbed and quinoa is fluffy. When quinoa is done, fluff with a fork and add parsley.

4. Mix quinoa and root vegetables. Serve warm.

Herbed Broiled Cod

Serve this Herbed Broiled Cod with a side of Quinoa Pilaf or Mexican Brown Rice (see recipes in Chapter 5).

INGREDIENTS | SERVES 2

1 tablespoon olive oil

1 tablespoon lemon juice

½ teaspoon dried dill

½ teaspoon dried parsley

½ teaspoon dried oregano

¼ teaspoon ground black pepper

¼ teaspoon salt

2 (6-ounce) cod fillets

1. Turn broiler on low.

2. Mix all ingredients except cod in a small bowl.

3. Place cod in a shallow baking dish and brush mixture on each fillet. Cook 5 minutes on each side or until fish flakes easily.

Two Servings of Fish Per Week Keeps the Doctor Away

Eating fish, like cod, at least twice per week can help reduce chronic inflammation, which has been associated with heart disease, type 2 diabetes, cognitive decline, Alzheimer's disease, osteoporosis, and depression.

Chicken Pesto with Brown Rice Ziti

The term "pesto" traditionally refers to a sauce made with basil, pine nuts, garlic, and olive oil that is typically served with pasta.

INGREDIENTS | SERVES 2

4 cups water

½ (16-ounce) package brown rice ziti

1½ cups chopped fresh basil

2 cloves garlic

⅓ cup pine nuts

½ cup plus 1 tablespoon olive oil

1 teaspoon salt, divided

1 teaspoon ground black pepper, divided

2 (4-ounce) boneless skinless chicken breasts, cut into cubes

1. Bring water to a boil in a saucepan over high heat. Add brown rice ziti and cook until al dente, about 8 minutes. Drain and set aside.

2. Combine basil, garlic, pine nuts, ½ cup olive oil, ½ teaspoon salt, and ½ teaspoon pepper in a food processor and pulse until smooth.

3. Heat remaining olive oil in a large skillet and add chicken. Season with remaining salt and pepper and cook until chicken is no longer pink, about 7–8 minutes.

4. When chicken is cooked, add cooked pasta and pesto sauce. Toss to combine. Serve warm.

Sprouted-Grain BLT

Technically, this recipe should be called a sprouted-grain BALT because of the addition of avocado, but you'll enjoy it so much, you won't even care.

INGREDIENTS | SERVES 2

6 slices nitrate-free turkey bacon

4 slices sprouted-grain bread

2 tablespoons Homemade Mayonnaise (see recipe in Chapter 10)

1 medium vine-ripened tomato, cut into slices

⅛ teaspoon salt

⅛ teaspoon ground black pepper

½ medium avocado, pitted, flesh removed, and sliced thinly

1. Cook bacon in a medium skillet over medium heat until crispy, about 3–4 minutes on each side. Place on paper towel and set aside.

2. Lightly toast bread. Spread 2 slices with 1 tablespoon mayonnaise each.

3. Top each mayonnaise-spread slice with half the tomato, salt, pepper, and avocado. Put 3 slices bacon on top of each stack. Finish off with remaining slices of bread. Serve immediately.

Chicken Salad with Walnuts and Cranberries

It may not be an easy feat to find unsweetened cranberries. Because they're so naturally tart, many manufacturers add sweeteners to make them more palatable. If you can't find unsweetened cranberries, use raisins or skip the dried fruit altogether.

INGREDIENTS | SERVES 2

2 slices sprouted-grain bread

1 (12.5-ounce) can shredded chicken breast

2 tablespoons Homemade Mayonnaise (see recipe in Chapter 10)

½ teaspoon salt

½ teaspoon ground black pepper

2 tablespoons chopped walnuts

¼ cup dried unsweetened cranberries

1. Lightly toast sprouted-grain bread.

2. Mix remaining ingredients in a medium bowl. Top each bread slice with half the chicken salad. Serve immediately.

A Note on Dried Fruit

Dried fruit should be considered a limited treat. Since all of the water content has been removed from the fruit, it's a fairly dense source of sugars and carbohydrates. Pay attention to amounts listed in recipes and don't overdo it on your portion sizes.

Tuna-Stuffed Avocado

Avocados serve as a creamy, cool vehicle for heart-healthy tuna in these stuffed avocado boats.

INGREDIENTS | SERVES 2

1 (5-ounce) can white tuna

2 tablespoons Homemade Mayonnaise (see recipe in Chapter 10)

2 hard-boiled large eggs, peeled and coarsely chopped

1 stalk celery, finely diced

1 tablespoon minced red onion

2 green onions, chopped

½ teaspoon salt

¼ teaspoon ground black pepper

1 medium avocado, halved, pitted, flesh removed whole

2 teaspoons hot sauce (optional)

1. Mix tuna, mayonnaise, eggs, celery, red and green onions, salt, and pepper together in a medium bowl.

2. Place half the tuna mixture in each avocado half. Top with hot sauce if desired.

But What about Mercury?

Tuna is often shunned because of its high mercury content. While it's true that you shouldn't overdo it on the mercury, tuna actually contains a special form of selenium, called selenoneine, that serves as an antioxidant that protects the fish's red blood cells from damage. Selenoneine is able to bind with the mercury compounds in the fish to reduce the risk of mercury-related problems.

Chicken Vegetable Stir-Fry

Try different variations of this recipe by using flank steak or skirt steak in place of chicken and switching up your vegetable choices.

INGREDIENTS | SERVES 2

1 cup brown rice

1½ cups water

¼ teaspoon coarse salt

2 tablespoons sesame oil

2 cloves garlic, minced

1 cup broccoli florets

4 asparagus stalks, cut into 2" pieces

½ cup matchstick carrots

½ cup bean sprouts

6 ounces boneless skinless chicken breasts, cut into cubes

2 tablespoons coconut aminos

2 tablespoons crushed almonds

Enzyme-Rich Sprouts

Bean sprouts are usually the sprouted version of the mung bean. They're often used in stir-frying because they're substantial enough to stand up to the high heat. Bean sprouts are especially rich in enzymes. In fact, it's estimated that sprouts contain 100 times more enzymes than unsprouted fruits and vegetables.

1. Combine rice, water, and salt in a medium saucepan over medium-high heat. Bring to boil and allow to boil 1 minute. Cover and reduce heat to low. Allow to simmer 20–25 minutes or until water is absorbed and rice is fluffy.

2. Heat sesame oil in a wok or medium skillet over high heat. Add garlic and sauté until fragrant, about 3 minutes. Add broccoli and asparagus and cook until tender, about 7 minutes, stirring frequently. Add carrots and sprouts and continue to cook until carrots are soft, about 4–5 minutes.

3. Add chicken and coconut aminos and cook until chicken is no longer pink, about 8 minutes.

4. Stir in almonds and remove from heat. Serve warm over rice.

Turkey, Sweet Potato, and Broccoli Bowls

These bowls are easy to throw together and get even better the day after cooking. Prepare a big batch in advance and divide it up into separate containers for lunch for the whole week.

INGREDIENTS | SERVES 4

2 medium sweet potatoes, peeled and diced

1 tablespoon olive oil

½ teaspoon coarse sea salt

1 head broccoli, cut into small florets (about 4 cups)

1 tablespoon coconut oil

½ pound ground turkey breast

1 teaspoon garlic powder

1 teaspoon onion powder

½ teaspoon salt

½ teaspoon ground black pepper

½ teaspoon ground sage

½ teaspoon fennel seed

¼ teaspoon red pepper flakes (optional)

1. Preheat oven to 400°F. Line a baking sheet with parchment paper.

2. In a large bowl, combine sweet potatoes, olive oil, and coarse salt and toss to combine. Spread out in a single layer on baking sheet and bake 25 minutes or until potatoes are soft and starting to brown. Flip once while cooking.

3. Steam broccoli in a double broiler until tender but still bright green, about 8 minutes.

4. Heat coconut oil in a large skillet over medium-high heat. Add turkey and cook about 4 minutes. Add remaining ingredients and continue cooking until turkey is no longer pink, about 4 more minutes.

5. Add sweet potatoes and broccoli to turkey and stir to combine. Remove from heat and allow to cool 5 minutes. Divide into serving bowls and serve warm.

Mediterranean Hummus Salad

The flavors of roasted red peppers and hummus in this Mediterranean salad complement each other perfectly.

INGREDIENTS | SERVES 2

4 tablespoons prepared hummus (no sugar added)

4 cups mixed greens

½ cup kalamata olives

½ cup chopped roasted red peppers

3 tablespoons minced red onion

½ cup canned chickpeas, drained and rinsed

Juice from ½ large lime

Juice from ½ large lemon

2 tablespoons olive oil

1 teaspoon Italian seasoning

1. Scoop 2 tablespoons hummus onto two serving plates. Top each plate with half the mixed greens, olives, red peppers, red onion, and chickpeas.

2. In a small bowl, whisk together lime juice, lemon juice, olive oil, and Italian seasoning. Drizzle dressing equally over each salad. Serve immediately.

I Can See Clearly Now

Roasted red peppers are rich in vitamin A, which promotes healthy night vision and can help prevent night blindness. They're also a vitamin C powerhouse, offering 300 percent of your daily needs for the day.

Baby Spinach and Avocado Salad

Baby spinach is a mild green that makes a great base for this salad, but you can also try kale, baby kale, mixed greens, or romaine lettuce.

INGREDIENTS | SERVES 1

2 cups baby spinach

¼ medium avocado, pitted, flesh removed, and sliced

¼ cup sliced strawberries

2 tablespoons sunflower seeds

2 tablespoons balsamic vinegar

2 tablespoons olive oil

1 teaspoon dried basil

⅛ teaspoon salt

⅛ teaspoon ground black pepper

1. Combine baby spinach, avocado, strawberries, and sunflower seeds in a medium bowl. Toss to combine.

2. In a separate small bowl, whisk together remaining ingredients. Pour over salad mixture and toss to coat. Let sit 3 minutes before serving to allow spinach to start to wilt.

Tuna Salad Roll-Up

You can switch up this basic tuna salad recipe by swapping the tuna for chicken or canned salmon or replacing some of the tuna with hard-boiled egg and making it a tuna and egg salad.

INGREDIENTS | SERVES 2

1 (5-ounce) can tuna in water

2 tablespoons Homemade Mayonnaise (see recipe in Chapter 10)

2 tablespoons chopped celery

1 tablespoon chopped scallions

¼ teaspoon salt

¼ teaspoon ground black pepper

2 sprouted-grain tortillas

1 cup baby spinach

¼ cup chopped roasted red peppers

2 teaspoons yellow mustard

1. Combine tuna, mayonnaise, celery, scallions, salt, and pepper in a medium bowl and mix until all ingredients are incorporated.

2. Scoop half the tuna mixture onto each tortilla and top each with ½ cup spinach, ⅛ cup roasted red pepper, and 1 teaspoon yellow mustard. Roll and secure with a toothpick.

CHAPTER 13

MD Stage 3 Dinner

Stuffed Sweet Potatoes

These stuffed sweet potatoes are so divine, you'll feel like you're being naughty even though you're not!

INGREDIENTS | SERVES 2

1 medium sweet potato, cut in half lengthwise

1 tablespoon coconut oil

½ pound lean ground beef

1 teaspoon garlic powder

1 teaspoon onion powder

½ teaspoon salt

¼ teaspoon ground black pepper

¼ teaspoon chili powder

1 cup chopped spinach

½ medium avocado, pitted, flesh removed, and sliced

¼ teaspoon chunky sea salt

Sweet Potato Starch Is Your Friend!

Because sweet potatoes are so starchy, many people think that they can't possibly be good for controlling blood sugar levels, but that couldn't be further from the truth. Sweet potatoes can actually improve blood sugar regulation—even in those with type 2 diabetes.

1. Preheat oven to 400°F.

2. Place sweet potato halves face-down on a baking sheet. Bake 25 minutes or until potatoes are soft.

3. While potatoes are cooking, heat coconut oil in a medium skillet over medium-high heat. Add ground beef and stir. When beef starts to brown, about 5 minutes, add garlic powder, onion powder, salt, pepper, and chili powder. Continue cooking ground beef until no longer pink, about 5 more minutes. Add chopped spinach and stir until wilted, about 3 minutes. Remove from heat.

4. When sweet potato is done cooking, remove from the baking sheet and mash the sweet potato flesh inside the skin. Top each sweet potato half with half the beef and spinach mixture, then add half the avocado to each potato and sprinkle with chunky sea salt.

5. Serve immediately.

Basil-Pesto Spaghetti Squash

*Replacing the chicken sausage in this recipe with some beans or chickpeas makes
this recipe vegetarian-friendly while preserving the protein content.*

INGREDIENTS | SERVES 4

1 (4-pound) spaghetti squash, top removed, halved lengthwise, and seeds removed

1 tablespoon olive oil

½ teaspoon sea salt

½ teaspoon ground black pepper

1 cup packed fresh basil leaves

1 clove garlic

¼ cup pine nuts

¼ cup olive oil

3 chicken sausage links (approximately 9 ounces), roughly chopped

1. Preheat oven to 400°F.

2. Place squash on baking sheet cut-side up. Brush with 1 tablespoon olive oil and then sprinkle with salt and pepper. Bake 40 minutes or until squash is tender.

3. Combine basil, garlic, pine nuts, and olive oil in a food processor and process until smooth. Set aside.

4. Cook sausage in a medium skillet over medium-high heat until browned on all sides, about 5 minutes.

5. Remove spaghetti squash from skin with a fork to create pasta-like strands. Toss with sausage and pesto until coated. Serve immediately.

Coconut Curry Salmon

The combination of curry, cumin, and ginger brings out the natural flavor of the salmon in this recipe. You can also try it with chicken instead.

INGREDIENTS | SERVES 2

2 teaspoons olive oil

½ cup chopped white onion

2 teaspoons curry powder

1 teaspoon ground cumin

½ teaspoon red pepper flakes

2 cups full-fat coconut milk

1 tablespoon fresh lime juice

2 teaspoons freshly grated ginger

1 tablespoon fish sauce

4 (4-ounce) salmon fillets

2 medium plum tomatoes, seeded and diced

1. Heat olive oil in a medium skillet over medium-high heat. Add onion, curry powder, cumin, and red pepper flakes. Sauté until onion is translucent, about 4 minutes.

2. Add coconut milk, lime juice, ginger, and fish sauce and bring to a boil. Reduce heat and simmer 5 minutes.

3. Add salmon, cover, and cook 6–8 minutes or until fish is cooked through.

4. Add tomatoes and toss in sauce. Serve immediately.

Choosing a Fish Sauce

When looking for a fish sauce, choose one that is gluten-free and made with minimal ingredients. Red Boat Fish Sauce is ideal because it's made with only freshly caught wild anchovies and natural sea salt.

Roasted Chicken with Carrots and Sweet Potatoes

As this chicken roasts, the flavor of the carrots and sweet potatoes merge with the chicken juice and oil to create an unbeatable sauce.

INGREDIENTS | SERVES 2

1 (3-pound) whole roasting chicken
3 tablespoons olive oil, divided
1 teaspoon dried thyme
2 teaspoons dried rosemary
2 teaspoons paprika
1 teaspoon salt, divided
2 cups diced sweet potatoes
2 cups chopped carrots
1 teaspoon ground cinnamon

1. Preheat oven to 350°F.

2. Put chicken in a roasting pan and rub with 2 tablespoons olive oil. Sprinkle thyme, rosemary, paprika, and ½ teaspoon salt on chicken.

3. Combine sweet potatoes, carrots, remaining olive oil, cinnamon, and remaining salt in a large bowl. Toss to coat. Arrange vegetables around chicken.

4. Bake 1 hour or until chicken reaches an internal temperature of 165°F.

5. Remove from heat and allow to cool slightly before serving.

Slow Cooker Roast Beef and Mushrooms

The best beef cuts for roasting include chuck, brisket, and round. Look for chuck roast, shoulder steak, brisket, rump roast, or bottom round.

INGREDIENTS | SERVES 4

½ cup dried minced onion
1 teaspoon onion powder
1 teaspoon garlic powder
½ teaspoon celery salt
1 teaspoon ground black pepper
1 teaspoon sea salt
1 (2.5-pound) beef roast
⅓ cup coconut aminos
2 cups sliced brown mushrooms

1. Combine minced onion, onion powder, garlic powder, celery salt, pepper, and sea salt in a small bowl. Rub spice mixture all over beef roast.

2. Place beef in a slow cooker with coconut aminos and mushrooms.

3. Cook on low 8–10 hours or high 5–6 hours.

Quinoa Soup

Quinoa is often served as a side dish, but it's the star of the show in this savory Quinoa Soup.

INGREDIENTS | SERVES 8

2 tablespoons olive oil

2 cloves garlic, minced

1 medium yellow onion, peeled and chopped

2 large carrots, peeled and chopped

2 stalks celery, chopped

10 cups vegetable broth

1 cup quinoa, rinsed and drained

1 (14.5-ounce) can petite diced tomatoes

1 (15-ounce) can cannellini beans, drained and rinsed

1 teaspoon garlic powder

1 teaspoon onion powder

1 tablespoon coconut aminos

1 teaspoon salt

½ teaspoon ground black pepper

1 teaspoon dried parsley

1 teaspoon paprika

3 bay leaves

¼ cup chopped cilantro, for garnish

1. In a large stockpot, heat olive oil over medium-high heat. Add garlic and sauté until fragrant, about 3 minutes. Add onion, carrots, and celery and continue to sauté until softened, about 5–6 minutes.

2. Add remaining ingredients except cilantro and bring to a boil. Reduce heat to low and simmer 90 minutes.

3. Top with cilantro before serving if desired.

The Gold of the Incas

Approximately 3,000 to 4,000 years ago, the Incas realized that quinoa was fit for human consumption, which is why the pseudograin has been nicknamed "the gold of the Incas." They believed it would increase the stamina of their warriors so that they were able to fight better. This increase in energy that comes from quinoa is due to its high riboflavin (or vitamin B_2 content). Riboflavin improves energy metabolism within brain and muscle cells.

Beet Soup

This beet soup is rich and creamy without any unhealthy ingredients.
Pair it with a salad for a well-balanced meal.

INGREDIENTS | SERVES 6

1 tablespoon olive oil
1 large yellow onion, peeled and diced
2 cloves garlic, minced
4 large beets, peeled and chopped
3 cups vegetable broth
1 (14.5-ounce) can full-fat coconut milk
½ teaspoon salt
¼ teaspoon ground black pepper

1. In a large stockpot, heat olive oil over medium heat. Add garlic and onion and sauté until translucent, about 4 minutes.

2. Add beets and broth and bring to a boil. Reduce heat to low and allow to simmer 25 minutes or until beets are fork tender.

3. Use an immersion blender to purée beets. Stir in remaining ingredients and serve warm.

The Crimson Power Food

Beets are one of the best sources of folate and betaine, two nutrients that work together to lower blood levels of homocysteine—an inflammatory compound that has the potential to damage your arteries and increase your risk of heart disease. The pigments that give beets their crimson color—called betacyanins—have also been shown to help fight cancer.

Slow Cooker Lentils and Sausage

You can use any variety of lentils for this soup, but red lentils tend to be the best texture for thickening soups since they get mushier than other varieties when cooked.

INGREDIENTS | SERVES 2

½ pound cooked spicy chicken sausage, cut into ¼"-thick medallions

4 cups vegetable broth

1 (15-ounce) can petite diced tomatoes

1 cup dried lentils, rinsed and drained

1 medium yellow onion, peeled and chopped

2 cups baby spinach leaves

2 cloves garlic, minced

½ teaspoon salt

Combine all ingredients in a slow cooker and cook on low 8 hours or until lentils are tender.

Lentils: A Nutrition-Packed Legume

Lentils have the highest amount of protein by weight of any other plant-based food. They're also low in fat and calories and compared to other legumes, like beans, and are a lot easier for your body to digest.

Curried Chicken Pita

If you can't find sprouted-grain pita bread, you can use sprouted-grain tortillas and turn this dinner into curried chicken wraps.

INGREDIENTS | SERVES 4

1 (15.5-ounce) can shredded chicken breast

2 tablespoons Homemade Mayonnaise (see recipe in Chapter 10)

1 teaspoon curry powder

1 tablespoon chopped green onions

1 teaspoon fresh lemon juice

4 (5") sprouted-grain pita breads, cut in half

1 cup alfalfa sprouts

1. Combine chicken, mayonnaise, curry powder, green onions, and lemon juice in a medium bowl and stir until incorporated.

2. Stuff mixture equally into each pita bread and top with sprouts.

The "Father of All Foods"

The word "alfalfa" is rooted in the Arabic word that translates to the "father of all foods." Traditionally, alfalfa was used to increase appetite and ease indigestion. Alfalfa sprouts are rich in vitamins A, C, and K and the minerals magnesium, iron, and calcium.

Tomato Basil Salmon

If you prefer, you can use chopped fresh tomatoes in place of fire-roasted diced tomatoes in this recipe.

INGREDIENTS | SERVES 2

2 (6-ounce) salmon fillets
¼ teaspoon sea salt
⅛ teaspoon ground black pepper
1 tablespoon dried basil
½ cup fire-roasted diced tomatoes, drained
2 teaspoons olive oil

1. Preheat oven to 375°F. Line a baking sheet with parchment paper.

2. Place salmon on baking sheet. Sprinkle salt, pepper, and basil on top of fish.

3. Spoon ¼ cup tomatoes over each fillet and drizzle each with 1 teaspoon olive oil.

4. Bake 20 minutes or until salmon flakes easily with a fork.

Spaghetti Squash with Kale and Chickpeas

You can make this spaghetti squash more appealing to the meat lover by adding some cooked cubed chicken breast or cooked ground beef or turkey.

INGREDIENTS | SERVES 2

1 (4-pound) spaghetti squash, top removed, halved lengthwise, and seeds removed

4 tablespoons olive oil, divided

½ teaspoon sea salt

¾ teaspoon ground black pepper, divided

2 cloves garlic, minced

1 (15-ounce) can chickpeas, drained and rinsed

3 cups chopped kale

½ teaspoon salt

½ cup toasted pine nuts

Superior to Spaghetti

Spaghetti squash gets its name from the fact that, when cooked, its flesh resembles strands of spaghetti. The squash is nutritionally superior to pasta, which is high in carbohydrates but low in other nutrients. Spaghetti squash is rich in vitamin A and the B vitamins niacin, folate, thiamine, and riboflavin.

1. Preheat oven to 400°F.

2. Place squash on baking sheet cut-side up. Brush with 1 tablespoon olive oil and then sprinkle with sea salt and ½ teaspoon pepper. Bake in oven 40 minutes or until squash is tender. Remove flesh in strands with a fork.

3. While squash is cooking, heat 2 tablespoons olive oil over medium-high heat in a skillet. Add garlic and sauté until fragrant, about 3 minutes.

4. Add chickpeas, kale, salt, and ¼ teaspoon pepper and continue to cook until kale wilts, about 4 minutes.

5. Add in spaghetti squash, pine nuts, and remaining olive oil and toss to combine. Serve immediately.

Spicy Lentil Wraps

If you don't have arrowroot powder, which is used as a thickener, you can use tapioca starch or tapioca flour in its place.

INGREDIENTS | SERVES 2

5 tablespoons white wine vinegar

2 cloves garlic, minced

1 small red chili pepper, seeded and minced

1 teaspoon arrowroot powder

1 teaspoon grated ginger

¾ teaspoon salt, divided

¼ teaspoon granulated stevia (optional)

1 tablespoon olive oil

1 medium yellow onion, peeled and chopped

1 teaspoon ground cumin

1 teaspoon chili powder

½ teaspoon red pepper flakes

¼ teaspoon cayenne pepper

½ cup dried lentils, rinsed and drained

2 cups vegetable broth

2 tablespoons chopped parsley

4 sprouted-grain tortillas

1. Combine vinegar, garlic, chili pepper, arrowroot, ginger, ¼ teaspoon salt, and stevia in a small saucepan over high heat and bring to a boil. Immediately reduce heat to low and cook another 2–3 minutes or until sauce thickens. Set aside.

2. Heat olive oil in a medium saucepan over medium heat. Add onions and cook until translucent, about 4 minutes. Add cumin, chili powder, red pepper flakes, cayenne, and ½ teaspoon salt and continue cooking 1 more minute.

3. Add lentils and broth to saucepan and bring to a boil. Cover, reduce heat to low, and simmer 20 minutes or until lentils are soft.

4. When lentils are done cooking, remove from heat and stir in parsley.

5. Put equal amounts lentil mixture in each tortilla and drizzle sauce on top.

Quinoa Taco Salad Bowls

Instead of building these quinoa tacos in a bowl, you can also wrap them in large lettuce, Swiss chard, or cabbage leaves.

INGREDIENTS | SERVES 6

1 cup quinoa, rinsed and drained

2 cups chicken broth

1 pound lean ground beef

1 (15-ounce) can black beans, drained and rinsed

1 tablespoon chili powder

1½ teaspoons ground cumin

1 teaspoon salt

1 teaspoon ground black pepper

½ teaspoon paprika

¼ teaspoon red pepper flakes

¼ teaspoon dried oregano

¼ teaspoon garlic powder

¼ teaspoon onion powder

1 cup chopped lettuce

1 cup salsa

½ cup sliced olives

¼ cup chopped cilantro

1 large avocado, pitted, flesh removed, and sliced thinly

1. Combine quinoa and broth in a medium saucepan. Bring to a boil over high heat and then reduce heat to low, cover, and allow to simmer 20 minutes or until broth is absorbed and quinoa is fluffy.

2. Heat a medium skillet over medium-high heat and add beef. Cook until no longer pink, about 10 minutes. Once beef is cooked, reduce heat to low and add beans and seasonings and stir until evenly coated.

3. Divide quinoa evenly between six bowls and top each bowl with equal amounts beef mixture, lettuce, salsa, olives, cilantro, and avocado.

Mediterranean Sweet Potatoes

*For some variation on this recipe, you could replace the sweet potatoes
with acorn squash or substitute white beans for the chickpeas.*

INGREDIENTS | SERVES 4

2 large sweet potatoes, cut in half lengthwise

1 (15-ounce) can chickpeas, drained and rinsed

3 teaspoons olive oil, divided

½ teaspoon ground cumin

½ teaspoon ground cinnamon

¼ teaspoon cayenne pepper

½ teaspoon smoked paprika

¼ teaspoon salt, divided

¼ cup tahini

1 tablespoon lemon juice

2 cloves garlic, minced

1 teaspoon minced jalapeño

¼ cup chopped tomatoes

¼ cup chopped roasted red peppers

¼ cup sliced black olives

¼ cup chopped cilantro

1. Preheat oven to 400°F and line two baking sheets with foil.

2. Place sweet potatoes face-down on baking sheet. Bake 30 minutes or until potatoes are soft.

3. On separate baking sheet, combine chickpeas, 2 teaspoons olive oil, cumin, cinnamon, cayenne, paprika, and ⅛ teaspoon salt. Toss to coat evenly and spread chickpeas out in a single layer on baking sheet. Bake 25–30 minutes or until just starting to crisp.

4. Combine tahini, lemon juice, garlic, jalapeño, and remaining olive oil and salt in a food processor and process until smooth.

5. Remove potatoes and chickpeas from oven. Mash potato flesh with a fork inside the potato skin. Top with roasted chickpeas, tomatoes, roasted red peppers, and black olives. Drizzle sauce over potatoes and top with fresh cilantro.

Asian Beef over Wild Rice

Wild rice bursts open when it's done cooking, so you'll be able to tell just by looking when the rice is finished.

INGREDIENTS | SERVES 4

1 cup wild rice

3 cups vegetable broth

3 tablespoons coconut aminos

2 tablespoons toasted sesame oil

¼ teaspoon salt

¼ teaspoon ground black pepper

1 tablespoon coconut oil

1 tablespoon freshly grated ginger

2 cloves garlic, minced

1 (1-pound) beef round, cut into 2" strips

1 cup sugar snap peas

¾ cup chopped carrots

Get Wild

Wild rice is actually a semiaquatic grass that grows in lakes, tidal rivers, and bays. Wild rice is higher in protein than other whole grains and is rich in fiber, folate, magnesium, zinc, and manganese. It's also rich in antioxidants.

1. Combine rice and broth in a medium saucepan and bring to a boil over high heat. Reduce heat to low and simmer covered 40–45 minutes or until rice kernels pop open and rice is tender.

2. In a small bowl, whisk together coconut aminos, sesame oil, salt, and pepper and set aside.

3. Heat coconut oil in a wok and add ginger and garlic. Sauté 1 minute and add sliced beef. Continue to cook until beef starts to brown, about 3 minutes. Add peas and carrots and continue to cook until almost tender, about 4 minutes. Add sauce mixture and bring to a boil. Reduce heat and allow to simmer 2–3 minutes.

4. Serve beef mixture over rice.

Lentil and Quinoa Chili

The combination of lentils and quinoa makes the chili a protein powerhouse—no meat necessary!

INGREDIENTS | SERVES 6

2 teaspoons coconut oil

2 cloves garlic, minced

1 small yellow onion, peeled and chopped

1 (15-ounce) can petite diced tomatoes

1 (15-ounce) can fire-roasted diced tomatoes

1 teaspoon ground cumin

1 tablespoon chili powder

1 teaspoon salt

½ teaspoon ground black pepper

3 cups vegetable broth

1 cup dried lentils, rinsed and drained

½ cup quinoa, rinsed and drained

1 (15-ounce) can dark red kidney beans, rinsed and drained

1 (15-ounce) can light red kidney beans, rinsed and drained

1. Heat coconut oil in a stockpot over medium-high heat. Add garlic and onion and sauté until fragrant, about 4 minutes.

2. Add tomatoes, cumin, chili powder, salt, and pepper and stir until combined. Add broth, lentils, and quinoa and bring to a boil. Reduce heat to low and simmer 45 minutes or until lentils are tender.

3. Stir in beans and simmer 5 more minutes. Serve warm.

Go Crazy over Coconut

Coconut is considered somewhat of an exotic food in the Western world, but it is a dietary staple in places like the South Pacific. Almost 50 percent of the fat in coconut is lauric acid, which is antibacterial, antiviral, and antifungal. Coconut oil in particular has been shown to reduce appetite, which can have a significant impact on weight loss.

Thai Noodle Bowl

You can make this recipe appropriate for Stage 2 by swapping out the brown rice pasta for strands of cooked spaghetti squash.

INGREDIENTS | SERVES 2

¼ cup coconut aminos

1 tablespoon toasted sesame oil

5 cups water, divided

½ teaspoon freshly grated ginger

2 cloves garlic, minced

¾ teaspoon granulated stevia

8 ounces brown rice pasta

2 tablespoons coconut oil

2 cups chopped broccoli

1 cup chopped cauliflower

2 medium carrots, peeled and cut into matchsticks

2 green onions, sliced thinly

½ cup bean sprouts

2 teaspoons sesame seeds

1. Combine coconut aminos, sesame oil, 1 cup water, ginger, garlic, and stevia in a small saucepan and stir over medium-low heat until heated through. Turn heat to low and allow to simmer 5 minutes. Set aside.

2. Bring 4 cups water to a boil in a large pot over high heat and add brown rice pasta. Cook 6–8 minutes or until pasta reaches desired level of doneness.

3. Heat coconut oil in a medium skillet over medium-high heat. Add broccoli, cauliflower, and carrots and sauté until starting to soften, about 8 minutes. Add green onions, sprouts, and sauce and continue cooking 5 minutes. Remove from heat, add pasta and sesame seeds, and toss to combine.

Sesame Oil: An Ayurvedic Staple

In Ayurvedic medicine, sesame oil is often used for its antibacterial and antifungal properties as well as its ability to fight inflammatory and cancer-causing processes.

Mexican Sweet Potato Casserole

You can put a spin on this recipe by adding some cooked ground beef or ground turkey and easing up on the beans.

INGREDIENTS | SERVES 6

1 tablespoon olive oil

1 cup quinoa, rinsed and drained

1 cup chicken broth

1 (15.5-ounce) can black beans, drained and rinsed

1 (15.5-ounce) can red kidney beans, drained and rinsed

1 (4-ounce) can green chilies

1 (15-ounce) can petite diced tomatoes

1 (15-ounce) can fire-roasted diced tomatoes

2 teaspoons chili powder

½ teaspoon cayenne pepper

1 teaspoon onion powder

½ teaspoon ground cumin

¼ teaspoon dried oregano

2 large sweet potatoes, peeled and diced

1 large avocado, pitted, flesh removed, and diced

½ cup sliced olives

1. Preheat oven to 350°F. Brush a 9" × 13" baking dish with olive oil.

2. Combine all ingredients except avocado and olives in baking dish and stir to combine. Spread out in dish and bake 60–90 minutes or until everything is cooked.

3. When casserole is done cooking, top with avocado and olives.

Stuffed Acorn Squash

When selecting an acorn squash, choose one that seems heavy for its size and is devoid of any soft spots or cracks in the skin. Store squash in a cool, dry place away from sunlight until ready to use.

INGREDIENTS | SERVES 4

2 small acorn squash, halved lengthwise and seeds removed

2 tablespoons olive oil, divided

½ medium yellow onion, peeled and diced

2 cloves garlic, minced

3 stalks celery, chopped

2 medium carrots, peeled and chopped

1 pound ground turkey

1 teaspoon salt

½ teaspoon ground black pepper

½ teaspoon ground sage

½ teaspoon dried thyme

2 cups chopped spinach

Boost Your Immunity

Although acorn squash grow in the winter, they actually belong to the class of summer squash, along with zucchini and yellow squash. Acorn squash is rich in dietary fiber as well as vitamin C, which helps boost the immune system by stimulating the production of white blood cells.

1. Preheat oven to 450°F.

2. Brush squash with 1 tablespoon olive oil and bake cut-side up on a baking pan for 30 minutes.

3. Heat remaining oil in a medium skillet over medium heat. Add onion and garlic and cook 4 minutes. Add celery and carrots and continue cooking until softened, about 5–6 minutes.

4. Add ground turkey, salt, pepper, sage, and thyme and continue cooking until turkey is no longer pink, about 8 minutes.

5. Add spinach and cook until wilted, about 3 minutes. Remove from heat.

6. Remove squash from oven and fill each "cup" with equal amounts beef mixture. Return squash to oven and continue cooking 30 more minutes.

Lentil and Sweet Potato Pita Pockets

This recipe calls for kale, but you can use your favorite dark leafy green.
Spinach, Swiss chard, collard greens, and beet greens also work well.

INGREDIENTS | SERVES 4

2 small sweet potatoes, peeled and cubed

2 tablespoons olive oil, divided

1 teaspoon coarse sea salt

1 small yellow onion, peeled and diced

2 cloves garlic, minced

1 teaspoon ground cumin

½ teaspoon ground cinnamon

½ teaspoon ground turmeric

½ teaspoon ground allspice

½ cup dried lentils, rinsed and drained

2 cups vegetable broth

2 cups chopped kale, ribs removed

4 sprouted-grain pita pockets, cut in half

An Anti-Inflammatory Effect

Curcumin—the main ingredient in turmeric—has powerful anti-inflammatory effects and is a strong antioxidant; however, curcumin is poorly absorbed into the bloodstream on its own. Pairing turmeric with black pepper, which contains piperine, can help enhance the absorption of curcumin by as much as 2,000 percent.

1. Preheat oven to 400°F. Line a baking sheet with parchment paper.

2. Put potatoes on baking sheet, drizzle with 1 tablespoon olive oil and sea salt, and toss to combine. Spread out in a single layer. Bake 25 minutes, flipping once while cooking.

3. While potatoes are cooking, heat remaining 1 tablespoon olive oil in a medium skillet over medium heat and add onion and garlic. Cook until translucent, about 4 minutes, then add cumin, cinnamon, turmeric, and allspice. Stir until combined.

4. Add lentils and broth to the skillet and bring to a boil. Reduce heat to low and allow to simmer 15 minutes.

5. Add kale to lentil mixture and simmer another 10 minutes until kale is wilted and lentils are soft.

6. Remove lentil mixture from saucepan, draining any excess liquid. When potatoes are done cooking, toss with lentils.

7. Stuff each pita pocket equally with the lentil mixture. Serve immediately.

MD Stage 3 Snacks and Sides

White Bean Hummus

Tahini is a paste made from ground sesame seeds. There are two types of tahini—hulled and unhulled. Unhulled tahini is the best choice because it's made from whole sesame seeds and therefore contains all of the nutrients.

INGREDIENTS | SERVES 6

1 (15.5-ounce) cans chickpeas, drained and rinsed

1 (15.5-ounce) can cannellini beans, drained and rinsed

½ cup tahini

3 tablespoons fresh lemon juice

1 teaspoon salt

1 clove garlic, minced

¼ teaspoon ground cumin

1 tablespoon olive oil

Put all ingredients in a food processor. Process until smooth.

Protein-Packed Sesame

Tahini has 20 percent complete protein, which makes it a higher protein source than most nuts and seeds. It's also easy to digest due to its high content of alkaline minerals, which are also beneficial in helping with weight loss.

Celery Boats

This upgraded snack is a twist on the classic "ants on a log," which uses peanut butter and raisins instead of cashew butter and coconut flakes.

INGREDIENTS | SERVES 2

4 stalks celery

4 tablespoons cashew butter

2 teaspoons coconut flakes

Fill each celery stalk with 1 tablespoon cashew butter. Sprinkle ½ teaspoon coconut flakes on top of each. Serve immediately.

Guacamole

*If you need a dose of healthy fat for any of the Stage 2 or Stage 3
recipes, just scoop a spoonful of this Guacamole on top.*

INGREDIENTS | SERVES 4

3 large avocados, halved, pitted, and flesh removed

Juice from 1 medium lime

2 medium Roma tomatoes, diced

2 cloves garlic, minced

¼ cup chopped cilantro

¼ cup chopped red onion

½ teaspoon salt

½ teaspoon ground black pepper

1 tablespoon diced jalapeño (optional)

1. Place avocado flesh and lime juice into a medium bowl and mash together with a fork, leaving some chunks intact.

2. Add tomatoes, garlic, cilantro, onion, salt, pepper, and jalapeño (if desired). Mash with a fork until combined.

Avocados Are More Than Healthy Fat

Avocados are rich in folate—a B vitamin that is associated with a lower risk of depression. Folate prevents an excess buildup of homocysteine—a compound that can interfere with the production of feel-good neurotransmitters like serotonin, dopamine, and norepinephrine and block nutrients from reaching the brain.

Green Beans with Almonds

For this recipe, choose raw slivered almonds. Roasted varieties often contain added salt, sugar, or refined oils.

INGREDIENTS | SERVES 4

6 cups water

1½ pounds green beans, trimmed and washed

2 tablespoons olive oil

½ cup slivered almonds

1 teaspoon minced garlic

¼ teaspoon salt

¼ teaspoon ground black pepper

Controlling Blood Sugar with Almonds

Almonds are naturally low in carbohydrates but rich in healthy fats, protein, and fiber, which makes them an ideal choice for diabetics or anyone else trying to control blood sugar levels. Almonds also contain a significant amount of magnesium. According to research, up to 38 percent of diabetics are deficient in magnesium, so consuming magnesium-rich foods and correcting the deficiency can lower blood sugar levels and improve the function of insulin.

1. Bring water to a boil in a large stockpot over high heat. Once water is boiling, reduce heat to medium-high and add green beans and cook until beans are soft but still crisp and bright green, about 3 minutes. Drain and rinse with cold water.

2. Heat olive oil in a medium skillet over medium heat. Add almonds and sauté 5 minutes or until lightly toasted. Transfer almonds to a paper-towel-lined plate with a slotted spoon.

3. Add garlic to oil in pan and sauté until fragrant, about 3 minutes. Toss green beans and almonds in pan along with salt and pepper. Mix until combined.

4. Remove from heat and serve immediately.

Turkey Bacon–Wrapped Asparagus

When choosing asparagus, look for bright green spears that have firm stems. Stems shouldn't be limp. If you buy asparagus in advance, cut off the bottoms and wrap the ends in a damp paper towel and store in the refrigerator in a plastic bag for up to 3 days.

INGREDIENTS | SERVES 4

6 slices nitrate-free turkey bacon (no sugar added), halved lengthwise

12 asparagus spears, ends trimmed

1. Wrap each bacon piece around each asparagus spear and secure in place with a toothpick.

2. Grill over medium heat 10 minutes or until bacon is crisp, turning each spear over halfway through cooking time.

Baked Mushrooms

White mushrooms are the most versatile of the mushroom varieties and can be used for almost any dish. Baby bella mushrooms have a more earthy flavor, but would work well in this side dish also.

INGREDIENTS | SERVES 2

1 teaspoon dried rosemary

1 teaspoon dried thyme

½ teaspoon salt

¼ teaspoon ground black pepper

1 tablespoon olive oil

1 tablespoon balsamic vinegar

2 cups whole white mushrooms

1. Preheat oven to 450°F. Line a baking sheet with parchment paper.

2. In a small bowl, whisk together rosemary, thyme, salt, pepper, olive oil, and vinegar.

3. Place the mushrooms cap-side down on baking sheet and brush olive oil mixture over each one, covering the mushrooms thoroughly.

4. Bake 15 minutes or until mushrooms are cooked through and starting to brown.

The Benefits of Balsamic Vinegar

Balsamic vinegar is a thick, syrup-like vinegar that is prepared by cooking grapes and letting the grape juice age for three to twelve years. The vinegar doesn't just add flavor; it has important health benefits. Balsamic vinegar contains polyphenols that stimulate the activity of pepsin—an enzyme that helps digest proteins. The polyphenols also help your intestines absorb amino acids.

Lemon Spinach Artichoke Dip

The cashews in this recipe make a surprisingly good replacement for the dairy that is in traditional spinach and artichoke dip.

INGREDIENTS | SERVES 2

2 (14-ounce) cans artichoke hearts in water
10 ounces frozen spinach
¾ cup cashews
2 tablespoons olive oil
1 tablespoon fresh lemon juice
1 clove garlic, minced
1 teaspoon onion powder
½ teaspoon salt
½ teaspoon ground black pepper

1. Combine artichoke hearts and frozen spinach in medium saucepan over medium heat.

2. While vegetables are warming up, put cashews in a food processor and process into a fine meal. Add olive oil, lemon juice, garlic, onion powder, salt, and pepper and process until smooth.

3. Once artichoke and spinach mixture is warm, drain excess liquid and pour cashew mixture into the saucepan. Stir over low heat until everything is incorporated. Serve warm.

Roasted Red Pepper Hummus

This Roasted Red Pepper Hummus is not only a great accompaniment for any cut-up vegetables, it also makes a delicious sandwich spread or salad dressing.

INGREDIENTS | SERVES 6

¼ cup tahini
3 tablespoons fresh lemon juice
1 (15-ounce) can chickpeas, drained and rinsed with liquid reserved
½ cup liquid from chickpeas
2 cloves garlic, minced
1 tablespoon olive oil
½ cup chopped roasted red peppers
½ teaspoon ground cumin
½ teaspoon salt

1. Combine tahini and lemon juice in a food processor and process 45 seconds. Stop and scrape down sides of food processor bowl and process another 45 seconds.

2. Add remaining ingredients and process 30 seconds. Scrape down sides of bowl and pulse another 30 seconds.

3. Put into a serving bowl and refrigerate until ready to serve.

Sweet Potato Fries

The goal with this recipe is to coat the sweet potato fries with oil without completely soaking them. You want them to be moist but not drenched, so reduce the amount of oil if necessary.

INGREDIENTS | SERVES 4

2 medium sweet potatoes, peeled and cut into 3" fries
1 tablespoon avocado oil
1 teaspoon sea salt
½ teaspoon ground cinnamon

Effective Fat-Soluble Vitamin Absorption

The combination of avocado oil and sweet potato in this recipe is a calculated one. Sweet potatoes are extremely high in vitamin A, which is a fat-soluble vitamin. Avocado oil is high in healthy fats, which help your body absorb the fat-soluble vitamins. Pairing these two powerhouses together can increase the absorption of the fat-soluble vitamins and antioxidants by as much as fifteen times.

1. Preheat oven to 400°F. Line a baking sheet with parchment paper.

2. Put potatoes on baking sheet, drizzle with avocado oil, and sprinkle sea salt and cinnamon on top. Toss potatoes, making sure to cover them with the mixture.

3. Spread out fries in a single layer on the baking sheet.

4. Bake 25 minutes or until fries are starting to brown, turning once while baking. Serve immediately.

Buffalo Hummus

Many buffalo-flavored dips are full of bad-for-you ingredients, but not this one.
You'll get the delicious satisfaction of spicy buffalo without any guilt.

INGREDIENTS | SERVES 4

1 (15-ounce) can garbanzo beans, drained and rinsed

1 clove garlic, minced

1 tablespoon olive oil

1 tablespoon lemon juice

1 tablespoon sesame oil

1 tablespoon tahini

⅓ cup buffalo wing sauce (no sugar added)

⅛ teaspoon salt

Put all ingredients in a food processor and process until smooth.

Kale Chips

These Kale Chips don't taste like potato chips, but they're able to satisfy that
craving for crunch while also contributing valuable nutrients to your day.

INGREDIENTS | SERVES 2

1 large bunch kale

2 tablespoons olive oil

1 teaspoon salt

½ teaspoon ground black pepper

Curly Kale

The most popular—and well-known—variety of kale is curly kale, which is dark green with ruffled leaves and thick, fibrous stalks. This type of kale can be rather tough with a peppery flavor profile, which makes it perfect for kale chips.

1. Preheat oven to 375°F. Line a baking sheet with parchment paper.

2. Rinse kale well and dry thoroughly with paper towels. Remove center ribs and break the leaves into bite-sized pieces.

3. Pour olive oil over kale and massage into leaves for about 2 minutes. Sprinkle with salt and pepper.

4. Spread kale on baking sheet and bake 10–15 minutes or until crisp, checking frequently.

Roasted Chickpeas

These savory Roasted Chickpeas can satisfy your craving for something salty and crunchy, but if you're looking for a sweet snack, you can roast them with some cinnamon, stevia, and coconut oil instead.

INGREDIENTS | SERVES 4

1 (15.5-ounce) can chickpeas, drained and rinsed
1 tablespoon olive oil
½ teaspoon cayenne pepper
½ teaspoon salt
½ teaspoon paprika

1. Heat oven to 450°F. Line a baking sheet with aluminum foil.

2. Put chickpeas on baking sheet and toss with olive oil and spices.

3. Spread out in a single layer and bake 30 minutes or until browned, turning chickpeas over once while baking.

Baked Onion Rings

If you can't find cashew meal easily at your local grocery store, you can make your own by pulsing whole raw cashews in the food processor until it reaches a coarse texture.

INGREDIENTS | SERVES 4

1 large red onion, peeled and cut into rings
¼ cup coconut flour
1¼ teaspoons salt, divided
¼ teaspoon ground black pepper
2 large eggs
¾ cup cashew meal
1 teaspoon garlic powder
1 teaspoon onion powder

1. Preheat oven to 350°F. Line a baking sheet with foil.

2. Separate the full rings into individual rings.

3. Combine coconut flour, ¼ teaspoon salt, and pepper on a shallow plate.

4. Whisk eggs in a shallow bowl.

5. Combine cashew meal, remaining salt, garlic powder, and onion powder on a separate shallow plate.

6. Dip each onion ring into coconut flour mixture, then egg wash, then cashew meal mixture, making sure to coat thoroughly. Place onion rings in a single layer on baking sheet.

7. Bake 30–35 minutes or until browned.

Call on Quercetin

Red onions are one of the best natural sources of quercetin, a bioflavonoid that has been shown to reduce the risk of stomach cancer, inhibit the replication of viruses, and reduce the formation of intestinal polyps. Quercetin is also an effective antifungal, antibacterial, and anti-inflammatory agent.

Mashed Cauliflower

This Mashed Cauliflower is an ideal low-carbohydrate substitute for mashed potatoes. When you add creamy coconut milk and chicken broth, you won't even notice the difference.

INGREDIENTS | SERVES 6

1 large head cauliflower, broken into florets

¾ cup chicken broth

¼ cup full-fat coconut milk

2 tablespoons avocado oil

½ teaspoon garlic salt

½ teaspoon salt

½ teaspoon ground black pepper

1. Steam florets in a double boiler until fork tender, about 8 minutes.

2. Remove from heat and transfer to a food processor. Add remaining ingredients and process until smooth.

Smooth Operator

Using a food processor will make this Mashed Cauliflower perfectly smooth and creamy. If you prefer a chunkier version, use a handheld mixer instead and stop beating when the cauliflower has reached its desired consistency.

Roasted Brussels Sprouts

These are not your mama's Brussels sprouts. The combination of sage and balsamic vinegar gives them a robust taste that will have you wondering why you hated them for so long.

INGREDIENTS | SERVES 4

1 pound Brussels sprouts, stems trimmed and halved

2 tablespoons olive oil

1 teaspoon salt

½ teaspoon ground black pepper

½ teaspoon ground sage

2 tablespoons balsamic vinegar

1. Preheat oven to 400°F.

2. Put all ingredients except vinegar in a baking dish and toss to combine. Bake 25 minutes or until Brussels sprouts are fork tender and starting to brown.

3. Drizzle with vinegar as soon as sprouts come out of the oven. Serve warm.

Roasted Cauliflower and Broccoli

Let the cauliflower and broccoli roast until the tips start to brown a bit. That will give the dish a nice "charred" taste that pairs well with grilled meats.

INGREDIENTS | SERVES 6

2 cups broccoli florets

2 cups cauliflower florets

2 tablespoons olive oil

2 cloves garlic, minced

¼ teaspoon salt

¼ teaspoon ground black pepper

1. Preheat oven to 425°F. Line a baking sheet with foil.

2. Put broccoli and cauliflower on baking sheet.

3. Drizzle olive oil over vegetables; add garlic, salt, and pepper and toss to coat.

4. Spread out in a single layer and bake 25 minutes or until vegetables are tender.

A Diet Staple

Over the years, broccoli has become the picture of the ultimate health food—and the cruciferous vegetable has earned its spot rightfully. Broccoli contains a compound called glucoraphanin, which the body turns into another compound called sulforaphane, which helps fight cancer. Broccoli is also low in calories and high in fiber, which aids in weight loss and helps controls blood sugar. One cup of broccoli contains the same amount of protein as one cup of rice with only half of the calories.

Garlicky Greens

Save time by buying a bag of green beans that has already been washed, cleaned, and trimmed for you.

INGREDIENTS | SERVES 4

½ pound green beans, trimmed
¼ cup olive oil
2 cloves garlic, minced
⅓ cup toasted pine nuts
16 ounces fresh spinach
¼ teaspoon salt
¼ teaspoon ground black pepper

1. Bring a large pot of water to a boil over medium-high heat. Add green beans and cook until fork tender, 4–5 minutes. Drain.

2. Heat olive oil in a medium skillet over medium heat. Add garlic and pine nuts and sauté 3 minutes or until pine nuts are lightly browned.

3. Transfer green beans to skillet; add spinach, salt, and pepper and sauté until spinach wilts, about 3 minutes.

Turkey and Avocado Roll-Ups

This is a simple snack that can be adjusted to fit your taste. Use roast beef or sugar-free ham in place of turkey, or sprinkle on some salt and pepper instead of garlic salt.

INGREDIENTS | SERVES 6

2 large avocados, halved and pitted
8 slices (6 ounces) deli turkey (no sugar added)
½ teaspoon garlic salt

1. Before removing the flesh, cut each avocado half into 4 equal-sized slices making 16 slices total. Then remove slices from the skin.

2. Cut each turkey slice in half. Wrap each half-slice turkey around each avocado slice.

3. Secure with a toothpick. Sprinkle with garlic salt. Serve immediately.

Tuna Salad and Cucumber Bites

You can make variations of this recipe by using shredded chicken or canned salmon in place of the tuna or using zucchini or celery sticks in place of the cucumber.

INGREDIENTS | SERVES 4

2 (5-ounce) cans tuna

2 hard-boiled large eggs, peeled and chopped

½ cup Homemade Mayonnaise (see recipe in Chapter 10)

½ teaspoon salt

½ teaspoon ground black pepper

1 medium cucumber, cut into rounds

1. Drain tuna and put in a medium bowl with chopped eggs, mayonnaise, salt, and pepper. Mash with a fork until combined.

2. Top each cucumber slice with tuna mixture.

Cool as a Cucumber

Cucumbers are composed of 96 percent water, so they don't just offer nutrients; they actually contribute to your water intake for the day. When you eat cucumber, the high water content helps flush out toxins and aids in weight loss. Cucumber is also cooling, so eating one has been shown to help reduce the pain from heartburn.

Fried Cauliflower "Rice"

When shredding the cauliflower, process it just enough to create rice-like pieces, but not too much that it begins to blend together. If you process it too long, it will turn into mashed cauliflower.

INGREDIENTS | SERVES 6

1 large head cauliflower, broken into florets (about 6 cups)
2 tablespoons olive oil
2 tablespoons sesame oil
4 cloves garlic, minced
2 green onions, chopped
2 tablespoons coconut aminos
½ teaspoon garlic salt
3 large eggs, beaten
1 large avocado, peeled, pitted, and sliced

1. Attach grating attachment to food processor. Turn on food processor to low and add cauliflower florets while food processor is running.

2. In a large wok or skillet, heat olive oil and sesame oil. Add minced garlic and sauté 3 minutes.

3. Add cauliflower and sauté another 5 minutes, stirring frequently until cauliflower is softened. Add green onions, coconut aminos, garlic salt, and eggs and toss until eggs are cooked.

4. Top with sliced avocado.

CHAPTER 15

MD Stage 3 Dessert

Peaches and Pistachios with Coconut

This dessert can satisfy a sweet tooth without a bunch of empty calories. Choose pistachios that are unsalted.

INGREDIENTS | SERVES 2

2 medium peaches, sliced into strips

2 teaspoons full-fat coconut milk

1 tablespoon chopped pistachios

2 teaspoons unsweetened coconut flakes

Place each sliced peach on a serving plate. Drizzle with coconut milk and sprinkle chopped pistachios and coconut flakes on top.

Go Nuts for Pistachio Nuts

Pistachios are the lowest-calorie nut, containing only 4 calories per nut. Their shells also make them more "diet-friendly" because it takes more work to break open each one and eat it. Pistachios are also loaded with potassium and vitamin B_6, which can boost your immune system and improve your mood.

Chocolate Avocado Mousse

This avocado mousse is extremely decadent and does not taste like avocado at all.

INGREDIENTS | SERVES 4

2 large ripe avocados, halved, pitted, and flesh removed

1 teaspoon liquid stevia

⅓ cup unsweetened cocoa powder

2 tablespoons unsweetened coconut milk

1 teaspoon vanilla extract

½ teaspoon ground chia seeds

2 tablespoons chopped almonds (optional)

1. Place avocado flesh in a food processor and process until smooth. Add remaining ingredients except almonds and process 1 more minute.

2. Transfer to serving bowls and refrigerate at least 30 minutes. Top with chopped almonds if desired before serving.

Fill Up on Fiber

An ounce of chia seeds contains 12 grams of carbohydrates, but 11 of those grams come from fiber, which doesn't raise blood sugar and therefore doesn't trigger an insulin response. Because chia seeds are about 40 percent fiber by weight, they are one of the best sources of fiber in the world.

Pear Sorbet

You can adjust this basic sorbet recipe to your liking by replacing the pears with a fruit of your choice—peaches make a suitable replacement.

INGREDIENTS | SERVES 2

4 cups cubed pears

2 tablespoons granulated stevia

1 tablespoon lime juice

1 tablespoon lemon juice

1. Put pears in a food processor and process until smooth. Add remaining ingredients and continue to process until incorporated.

2. Pour mixture into a freezer-safe container and freeze 4 hours or until set.

Quinoa Pudding

Step out of your comfort zone by having quinoa for dessert instead of dinner. This quinoa pudding is a play on bread pudding but without the wheat.

INGREDIENTS | SERVES 8

1 cup quinoa, rinsed and drained

4 cups water

2 large eggs

2 large egg whites

1 cup full-fat coconut milk

1 teaspoon vanilla extract

1½ tablespoons granulated stevia

⅛ teaspoon salt

¼ teaspoon ground cinnamon

1. Preheat oven to 350°F.

2. Mix quinoa and water together in a medium saucepan and bring to a boil. Reduce heat and simmer uncovered 15 minutes. Drain quinoa with a cheesecloth, making sure to get rid of any excess water.

3. In a large mixing bowl, whisk together remaining ingredients. Stir in quinoa and mix until combined.

4. Pour batter into a greased 8" × 8" pan and bake 40 minutes or until a toothpick inserted in the center comes out clean. Serve warm.

Coconut Macaroons

These Coconut Macaroons are easy to whip up and contain protein that can actually keep you feeling full through the night until breakfast the next morning.

INGREDIENTS | SERVES 2

4 large egg whites

2 tablespoons granulated stevia

1 teaspoon almond extract

2 cups unsweetened grated coconut

The Incredible, Edible Egg White

Egg whites, which are low in calories and devoid of fat, contain the bulk of an egg's protein. A single egg white contains 4 grams of protein and only 17 calories.

1. Preheat oven to 375°F. Line a baking sheet with parchment paper.

2. Combine egg whites and stevia in a clean, medium mixing bowl and beat with a handheld mixer until stiff peaks form.

3. Fold in almond and coconut and gently mix to combine.

4. Drop coconut mixture onto baking sheet by spoonfuls.

5. Bake 15–20 minutes or until cookies are set and golden brown. Transfer to a wire rack and allow to cool before serving.

Almond Mug Cake

You can turn this Almond Mug Cake into a coconut mug cake by replacing the almond milk with coconut milk, removing the almond extract, and replacing the crushed almonds with coconut shavings.

INGREDIENTS | SERVES 1

3 tablespoons coconut flour
¼ teaspoon baking powder
⅔ teaspoon granulated stevia
¼ cup almond milk
¾ teaspoon melted coconut oil
½ teaspoon vanilla extract
¼ teaspoon almond extract
1 tablespoon crushed almonds

1. Whisk all ingredients together in a microwave-safe mug, making sure to thoroughly combine.

2. Microwave on high 90 seconds or until a toothpick inserted into center of cake comes out clean. Allow to cool slightly before serving.

Hidden Zucchini Brownies

These brownies are a good way to sneak some greens into your dessert—zucchini is so light, you won't even taste it.

INGREDIENTS | SERVES 2

1 cup unsweetened almond butter
1½ cups shredded zucchini
1 large egg
1 teaspoon vanilla extract
1 teaspoon baking soda
1½ teaspoons ground cinnamon
1 teaspoon liquid stevia

1. Preheat oven to 350°F.

2. Combine all ingredients together in a large mixing bowl and stir until evenly incorporated. Pour mixture into a greased 8" × 8" pan.

3. Bake 45 minutes or until brownies are set and a toothpick inserted in the center comes out clean.

Pumpkin Pie Mousse

*Cinnamon is made from the inner bark of trees of the Cinnamomum genus.
There are two main types: Ceylon cinnamon (often called "true cinnamon")
and cassia cinnamon (which is the more common variety today).*

INGREDIENTS | SERVES 2

1½ cups pumpkin purée
3 large eggs
1½ tablespoons granulated stevia
½ teaspoon salt
1 teaspoon ground cinnamon
1 teaspoon pumpkin pie spice
¼ teaspoon ground nutmeg
¾ cup full-fat coconut milk

1. Preheat oven to 350°F.

2. Whisk all ingredients together in a large mixing bowl. Pour mixture into a greased 8" × 8" baking pan.

3. Bake 30–40 minutes or until a toothpick inserted into the center comes out clean.

4. Refrigerate until cool. Serve chilled.

Sprinkle on the Cinnamon

Cinnamon can drastically reduce insulin resistance—a condition characterized by a high blood sugar levels and a decreased sensitivity to insulin. Insulin resistance often precedes diabetes. Cinnamon can also help directly lower blood sugar by interfering with the digestive enzymes that break down carbohydrates and slowing their release into the bloodstream.

Chocolate Coffee Mug Cake

If you don't have coffee-flavored extract, you can use a tablespoon of instant coffee granules instead or skip the coffee flavor altogether.

INGREDIENTS | SERVES 1

3 tablespoons blanched almond flour

2 tablespoons unsweetened cocoa powder

1/3 teaspoon granulated stevia

1 tablespoon unsweetened almond milk

1 teaspoon coconut oil, melted

1 teaspoon vanilla extract

1 large egg

1/8 teaspoon salt

2 drops coffee-flavored extract

1 teaspoon unsweetened almond butter

1. Beat all ingredients together with a fork in a microwave-safe mug. Microwave on high 2–3 minutes or until cake is set and toothpick inserted in center comes out clean.

2. Allow to cool 1–2 minutes before serving.

Blueberry Quinoa Pudding

This quinoa pudding makes a great dessert, but you can also enjoy it for breakfast. You can heat up the leftovers on the stove and eat them before heading out for the day.

INGREDIENTS | SERVES 4

3 cups unsweetened almond milk

¼ cup water

2 teaspoons vanilla extract

½ tablespoon granulated stevia

¼ teaspoon ground cinnamon

1 cup quinoa, rinsed and drained

½ cup blueberries

2 tablespoons chopped walnuts

1. Combine milk, water, vanilla, stevia, and cinnamon in a medium saucepan and stir over medium heat. Bring to a simmer and then stir in quinoa. Reduce heat to low and cook 30 minutes, stirring frequently.

2. Remove from heat and stir in blueberries and walnuts. Serve immediately.

Quinoa for Dessert

Quinoa makes a great dessert food because it's high in protein, which can help boost metabolism and significantly reduce appetite. It's also high in fiber, so when you're finished with your quinoa pudding, you'll actually feel full instead of just craving more. It also has a low glycemic index, so it won't significantly spike your blood sugar before heading off to bed.

Coconut Lime Mug Cake

You can turn this Coconut Lime Mug Cake into a coconut lemon cake by replacing the lime zest with some fresh lemon zest and adding a dash of lemon extract.

INGREDIENTS | SERVES 1

3 tablespoons coconut flour

4 tablespoons full-fat coconut milk

¼ teaspoon baking powder

⅔ teaspoon granulated stevia

1 teaspoon unsweetened shredded coconut

¼ teaspoon lime zest

1. Combine coconut flour, coconut milk, baking powder, and stevia in a microwave-safe mug and whisk until everything is incorporated. Stir in coconut and lime zest.

2. Microwave on high 90 seconds or until cake is set and toothpick inserted in center comes out clean. Allow to cool slightly before serving.

Blueberry Granita

This Blueberry Granita is easy to throw together. It's perfect for the summertime when fresh berries are plentiful and you need a dessert that can help cool you down.

INGREDIENTS | SERVES 2

2 cups fresh blueberries

1 tablespoon lemon juice

⅔ teaspoon granulated stevia

1 cup ice

1. Combine all ingredients in a blender and blend until smooth.

2. Pour mixture into an 8" × 8" baking dish and freeze 30 minutes.

3. After 30 minutes, scrape baking dish with a fork to create a slush. Return to freezer 1 hour then serve immediately.

Start Your Day with Lemon

Lemon juice contains pectin, a soluble fiber that has been shown to aid in weight loss. Lemon juice stimulates your digestive tract and helps with constipation. In addition to adding lemon juice to your dishes, try drinking fresh lemon juice in some warm water to start each day.

Raspberry Mug Cake

You can make this cake your own by swapping the fresh raspberries for any Stage 3–approved fruit of your choice.

INGREDIENTS | SERVES 1

1 large egg
2 tablespoons coconut cream
1 tablespoon melted coconut oil
⅛ teaspoon baking powder
⅛ teaspoon vanilla extract
1 teaspoon granulated stevia
5 tablespoons almond flour
¼ cup fresh raspberries

1. Mix egg, coconut cream, coconut oil, baking powder, vanilla, stevia, and flour in a microwave-safe mug until combined. Fold in raspberries.

2. Microwave on high 2 minutes or until cake is set and toothpick inserted in center comes out clean. Allow to cool slightly before serving.

Coffee Brownies

For this recipe, choose a raw dark chocolate cocoa powder that contains no added sugar. You want the type of cocoa that you bake with.

INGREDIENTS | SERVES 2

1 cup coconut cream

3 large eggs

1 teaspoon liquid stevia

1 cup crushed walnuts

¼ cup unsweetened cocoa powder

1 tablespoon instant coffee granules

1½ teaspoons vanilla extract

½ teaspoon baking soda

¼ teaspoon salt

¼ cup coconut oil, melted

1. Preheat oven to 325°F.

2. In a medium mixing bowl, combine all ingredients except coconut oil and stir until combined. Pour batter into a greased 9" × 13" baking pan.

3. Bake 25–30 minutes or until brownies are set and toothpick inserted in center comes out clean.

4. Remove from oven and drizzle melted coconut butter on top. Allow to cool before serving.

Is Chocolate a Health Food?

You've heard the studies about how great chocolate is for you, but that doesn't mean you can just freely eat chocolate bars whenever the urge strikes. The benefits of chocolate come from the raw cocoa, not the added sugar and other ingredients. Raw cocoa is packed with antioxidants that help destroy the free radicals that contribute to disease and premature aging.

Lemon Bars

If you don't have tapioca flour, you can use arrowroot starch in its place; just make sure to divide the amount in half, as they don't substitute one for one.

INGREDIENTS | SERVES 6

2 cups almond flour
¼ cup plus 2 tablespoons tapioca flour
¼ teaspoon baking soda
¼ teaspoon salt
½ tablespoon granulated stevia
½ teaspoon vanilla extract
½ cup coconut oil
2 large eggs
½ teaspoon liquid stevia
¼ cup fresh lemon juice
½ teaspoon lemon zest

Breaking Down Tapioca Flour

Tapioca flour is made from the starchy root vegetable called cassava or yucca. It's not very nutrient-dense, but it's hypoallergenic and acts as an excellent thickener and creates a "fluffiness" in gluten-free baked foods that you wouldn't be able to achieve with almond flour or coconut flour alone.

1. Preheat oven to 325°F.

2. Combine almond flour, ¼ cup tapioca flour, baking soda, salt, stevia powder, vanilla, and coconut oil in a medium mixing bowl and mix until completely incorporated.

3. Press mixture in the bottom of a greased 8" × 8" pan and bake 30 minutes or until crust starts to brown.

4. While crust is baking, beat eggs, liquid stevia, lemon juice, lemon zest, and remaining 2 tablespoons tapioca flour in a medium bowl. Pour mixture over baked crust and continue to bake 15–20 minutes or until set.

5. Allow to cool completely before serving.

Pumpkin Blondies

Blondies are the vanilla version of chocolate brownies. This blondie recipe has the added bonus of puréed pumpkin, which not only makes the flavor divine, but also adds several beneficial nutrients, like vitamin A.

INGREDIENTS | SERVES 2

2 cups almond flour
½ cup ground flaxseed
1 tablespoon granulated stevia
½ teaspoon salt
2 teaspoons almond extract
1 cup pumpkin purée
1 large egg

1. Preheat oven to 350°F.

2. In a medium mixing bowl, combine almond flour, flaxseed, stevia, and salt.

3. In a large bowl, mix almond extract, pumpkin purée, and egg until combined.

4. Fold dry ingredients into wet ingredients until just combined. Do not overmix. Pour into a greased 8" × 8" pan.

5. Bake 20–25 minutes or until blondies are set and toothpick inserted in center comes out clean.

Cashew Butter Bites

These Cashew Butter Bites are full of healthy fats and protein that will fill you up and keep you satisfied for the rest of the night. Take a couple along with you in the morning to snack on during the day.

INGREDIENTS | SERVES 6 (MAKES 12 BITES)

⅓ cup unsweetened cashew butter
1 tablespoon coconut oil
2 teaspoons vanilla extract
12 drops liquid stevia
¾ cup almond flour
1 tablespoon flaxseed

1. Mix all ingredients together in a medium bowl until thoroughly combined. Roll into 1" balls and place each ball on a parchment-paper-lined baking sheet.

2. Refrigerate 1 hour.

Cancer-Fighting Cashews

Cashews are rich in magnesium—the "relaxation mineral." Magnesium has been shown to reduce the frequency of migraines, help lower blood pressure, and improve cognitive ability. Proanthocyanidins—compounds that inhibit the multiplication and division of cancer cells—are also found in cashews.

Vanilla Mug Cake

This Vanilla Mug Cake is a great basic recipe that you can dress up with some fresh fruit, cacao nibs, coconut cream, or crushed nuts.

INGREDIENTS | SERVES 1

1 large egg
1 tablespoon coconut flour
1 tablespoon almond flour
1 teaspoon vanilla extract
⅔ teaspoon granulated stevia

1. Beat egg in a microwave-safe mug. Add remaining ingredients and whisk with a fork until combined.

2. Microwave 60–90 seconds or until cake is set. Allow to cool slightly before serving.

Chocolate Pudding

This healthy pudding is a chocolate lover's dream. It's best when eaten right away, but you can store any leftovers in the refrigerator and thin it out with some extra coconut milk before serving.

INGREDIENTS | SERVES 2

1 large egg

½ large avocado, pitted and flesh removed

¼ cup coconut milk

¼ teaspoon granulated stevia

2½ tablespoons unsweetened cocoa powder

1 tablespoon instant coffee granules

1 tablespoon coconut flour

⅛ teaspoon salt

2 tablespoons unsweetened coconut flakes

1. Add egg, avocado, and coconut milk to a food processor and process until smooth.

2. Add all remaining ingredients except coconut flakes and process again until smooth.

3. Transfer to two serving dishes and sprinkle coconut flakes on top.

Lemon Shortcake

*Turn this dessert into a berry shortcake by adding some fresh raspberries
and then topping with a scoop of whipped coconut cream.*

INGREDIENTS | SERVES 1

1 large egg

½ tablespoon coconut oil, melted

2 teaspoons unsweetened almond milk

¼ teaspoon lemon extract

¼ teaspoon lemon zest

2 teaspoons fresh lemon juice

1 tablespoon coconut flour

¼ teaspoon granulated stevia

½ teaspoon baking powder

1. Beat egg in a medium bowl. Add melted coconut oil, almond milk, lemon extract, lemon zest, and lemon juice and whisk until combined.

2. In a small bowl, mix together coconut flour, stevia, and baking powder. Fold into lemon mixture.

3. Pour into a mug and microwave 90 seconds or until cake is set. Allow to cool slightly before serving.

Arm Yourself with Almond Milk

Almond milk is low in carbohydrates, so it doesn't raise your blood sugar levels significantly like dairy milk does. It's also lower in calories, so it's perfect for adding to desserts.

Coconut Lime Popsicles

These popsicles are ready in a flash. You can mix up the flavor profile by adding lemon juice instead of lime or puréeing some berries and mixing them with coconut milk and stevia before freezing.

INGREDIENTS | SERVES 2

1½ cups full-fat coconut milk
1 teaspoon granulated stevia
2 tablespoons fresh lime juice

1. Whisk all ingredients together in a medium bowl. Taste mixture and adjust stevia or lime juice to taste.

2. Pour mixture into popsicle molds and freeze until solid.

Coconut Dip with Berries

This dessert is light and fresh and easy to throw together at a moment's notice. You can substitute other Stage 3–approved fruits in place of the berries.

INGREDIENTS | SERVES 2

1 (13.6-ounce) can full-fat coconut milk
1 teaspoon granulated stevia
¼ teaspoon vanilla extract
Juice of ½ large lemon
1 cup mixed berries (fresh or frozen)

1. Refrigerate coconut milk for at least 8 hours. When coconut milk is thoroughly chilled, scoop out the cream that forms on top of the liquid.

2. Put cream in a medium bowl and beat with a handheld mixer 3 minutes. Fold in stevia and vanilla.

3. Squeeze lemon juice on top. Scoop over berries.

Mixed-Berry Cobbler

This berry cobbler is made right in a single-serving, microwaveable-safe dish, which means no dishes and no leftovers to tempt you later in the evening.

INGREDIENTS | SERVES 1

¾ cup mixed blueberries, blackberries, and raspberries

2 teaspoons granulated stevia, divided

⅓ cup coconut flour

½ teaspoon baking powder

1 tablespoon coconut oil

2 tablespoons coconut milk

1. Combine berries and 1 teaspoon stevia in a mug and stir to mix. Let sit 5 minutes so berries can sweat.

2. Meanwhile, combine remaining stevia, coconut flour, and baking powder in a medium bowl and stir to combine. Cut in coconut oil and then mash in milk with a fork.

3. Place flour mixture on top of berries. Microwave on high 90 seconds or until topping is cooked.

4. Allow to cool before serving.

Chia Seed Pudding

As this Chia Seed Pudding sits in the refrigerator, the chia seeds will absorb the liquid and start to give the pudding a gelatinous consistency. If the pudding becomes too thick for your taste, stir in a little more almond milk right before eating.

INGREDIENTS | SERVES 4

½ cup raspberries

1½ cups unsweetened almond milk

⅓ cup chia seeds

¼ cup unsweetened cocoa powder

1 teaspoon granulated stevia

¼ teaspoon salt

½ teaspoon vanilla extract

1. Put raspberries in a food processor and process until puréed.

2. Mix all ingredients except raspberries in a medium mixing bowl and whisk to combine. Pour into four glass jars and top each equally with raspberry purée.

3. Refrigerate at least 4 hours or until pudding sets. Serve chilled.

Ch-Ch-Ch-Chia!

Due to their extremely high fiber content, chia seeds can hold multiple times their weight in water. This causes chia seeds to pull in water and expand in the stomach, which slows the absorption of food and makes you feel fuller longer.

Quinoa Bites

These Quinoa Bites are a great dessert, but they also make a wonderful midday snack that you can store in your car or at your desk at work and quickly grab on the go.

INGREDIENTS | SERVES 12

1 cup cooked quinoa
1 cup old-fashioned oats, uncooked
½ cup unsweetened coconut flakes
½ cup chopped peaches
1 teaspoon ground cinnamon
½ teaspoon ground nutmeg
¼ teaspoon salt
⅔ teaspoon granulated stevia
2 large eggs

Protect Your Brain with Nutmeg

Nutmeg contains a natural organic compound called myristicin, which is known to protect your brain against degenerative diseases such as Alzheimer's. Nutmeg also aids in sleep and has antibacterial properties that can help protect the teeth and gums from decay and disease.

1. Preheat oven to 350°F. Grease a mini-muffin tin.

2. In a large mixing bowl, combine quinoa, oats, coconut, and peaches.

3. In a small bowl, combine cinnamon, nutmeg, salt, and stevia. Fold spice mixture into quinoa mixture.

4. Lightly beat eggs in a small bowl and mix into quinoa mixture, stirring just until combined.

5. Scoop spoonfuls of the mixture into mini-muffin tin and bake 15–20 minutes or until bites are set and slightly golden.

Food Lists

Excluded from All Stages

Grains/Starches
Barley
Corn
Rye
Wheat
Other gluten-containing grains

Dairy Products
All (milk, yogurt, cheese, sour cream, ice cream)

Other
Processed foods
Refined sugar
Alcohol

Stage 1 Included Foods

Protein Sources
Beans
Beef
Buffalo
Chicken, boneless/skinless
Chickpeas (garbanzo beans)
Deli meats, nitrate- and sugar-free
Eggs
Fish and shellfish
Lentils/legumes
Pork
Turkey
Turkey bacon

Grains/Starches
Amaranth
Arrowroot
Baking powder
Brown rice (crackers, pasta, tortillas)
Millet

Oats, steel-cut only
Quinoa
Rice milk, unsweetened
Sprouted-grain breads
Tapioca
Wild rice

Fruits
All (with the exception of dried fruits)

Vegetables
All

Fats
None

Condiments/Spices
Broths
Coconut aminos
Dried and fresh herbs

Extracts (vanilla, almond, orange, coffee)
Garlic
Ginger
Horseradish
Ketchup
Mustard

Pickles
Salsa
Seasonings (no artificial ingredients)
Stevia (all forms)
Tomato paste
Vinegar (all types)

Stage 2 Included Foods

Protein Sources
Beans
Beef
Buffalo
Chicken, boneless/skinless
Chickpeas (garbanzo beans)
Deli meats, nitrate- and sugar-free
Eggs
Fish and shellfish
Pork
Turkey
Turkey bacon

Fruits
Lemon
Lime

Vegetables
Arugula
Artichokes
Asparagus
Beet greens
Broccoli
Brussels sprouts
Cabbage
Cauliflower
Celery
Collard greens

Cucumbers
Endive
Eggplant
Fennel
Green beans
Green chilies
Jicama
Kale
Leeks
Lettuce
Mushrooms
Mustard greens
Nori wraps/seaweed
Onions (red, yellow, green, and white)
Peppers
Shallots
Spinach
Spirulina
Sugar snap peas/peas
Swiss chard
Tomatoes
Watercress
Zucchini

Healthy Fats
Avocado
Avocado oil
Chia seeds

Coconut (oil, flakes, milk)
Flaxseed
Hummus
Mayonnaise, homemade
Nuts and seeds
Nut and seed butters
Nut and seed milks
Olive oil
Olives
Sesame seed oil
Tahini

Grains/Starches
None

Condiments/Spices
Broths
Coconut aminos
Dried and fresh herbs
Extracts (vanilla, almond, orange, coffee)
Garlic
Ginger
Horseradish
Mayonnaise, homemade
Mustard
Pickles
Salsa
Seasonings (no artificial ingredients)
Stevia (all forms)
Tomato paste
Vinegar (all types)

Stage 3 Included Foods

Protein Sources
Beans
Beef
Buffalo
Chicken, boneless/skinless
Chickpeas (garbanzo beans)
Deli meats, nitrate- and sugar-free
Eggs
Fish and shellfish
Lentils/legumes
Pork
Turkey
Turkey bacon

Fruits
Apples
Berries
Cherries

Cranberries
Grapefruit
Lemons
Limes
Peaches
Pears
Plums

Vegetables
All

Healthy Fats
Avocado
Avocado oil
Chia seeds
Coconut (oil, flakes, milk)
Flaxseed
Hummus

Mayonnaise, homemade
Nuts and seeds
Nut and seed butters
Nut and seed milks
Olive oil
Olives
Sesame seed oil
Tahini

Grains/Starches
Arrowroot powder
Baking powder
Brown rice (crackers, pasta, tortillas)
Oats (steel-cut and old-fashioned)
Quinoa
Sprouted-grain breads
Tapioca
Wild rice

Condiments/Spices
Broths
Coconut aminos
Dried and fresh herbs
Extracts (vanilla, almond, orange, coffee)
Garlic
Ginger
Horseradish
Mustard
Pickles
Salsa
Seasonings (no artificial ingredients)
Stevia (all forms)
Tomato paste
Vanilla (and other) extracts
Vinegar (all types)

Meal Plans

Week 1

Monday (Stage 1)
Breakfast: Apple-Cinnamon Quinoa Porridge
(Chapter 2)
Lunch: Open-Faced Turkey Sandwich (Chapter 3)
Dinner: Shrimp Skewers with Mango Salsa
(Chapter 4) and Mexican Brown Rice (Chapter 5)
Snack: Fruit Salad (Chapter 5)
Dessert: Strawberry Mug Cake (Chapter 6)

Tuesday (Stage 1)
Breakfast: Peach Pear Smoothie (Chapter 2)
Lunch: Taco Bowls (Chapter 3)
Dinner: Pulled Pork with Sweet Potatoes
(Chapter 4)
Snack: Roast Beef and Pickle Wraps (Chapter 5)
Dessert: Berry Salad with Cacao Nibs (Chapter 6)

Wednesday (Stage 1)
Breakfast: Overnight Oats (Chapter 2)
Lunch: Massaged Kale and Apple Salad
(Chapter 3)
Dinner: Slow Cooker Cilantro Lime Chicken
(Chapter 4) and Red Beans and Rice (Chapter 5)
Snack: Baked Grapefruit (Chapter 5)
Dessert: Blueberry-Poached Apples (Chapter 6)

Thursday (Stage 2)
Breakfast: Egg White Scramble (Chapter 7)
Lunch: Baked Meatballs (Chapter 8)

Dinner: Slow Cooker Pulled Pork Chili
(Chapter 9)
Snack: Smoked Salmon Bites (Chapter 10)

Friday (Stage 2)
Breakfast: Denver Omelet (Chapter 7)
Lunch: Eggplant Pizza (Chapter 8)
Dinner: Blackened Salmon (Chapter 9)
Snack: Spiced Nuts (Chapter 10)

Saturday (Stage 3)
Breakfast: Coconut Oatmeal (Chapter 11)
Lunch: Almond-Crusted Cod (Chapter 12)
Dinner: Stuffed Sweet Potatoes (Chapter 13)
Snack: Celery Boats (Chapter 14)
Dessert: Chocolate Avocado Mousse
(Chapter 15)

Sunday (Stage 3)
Breakfast: Vegetable-Packed Scrambled Eggs
(Chapter 11)
Lunch: Chicken Fajitas (Chapter 12)
Dinner: Basil-Pesto Spaghetti Squash
(Chapter 13)
Snack: Kale Chips (Chapter 14)
Dessert: Pear Sorbet (Chapter 15)

Week 2

Monday (Stage 1)
Breakfast: Spirulina Power Smoothie (Chapter 2)
Lunch: Hearty Lentil Soup (Chapter 3)

Dinner: Seared Scallop Salad (Chapter 4) and Smashed Sweet Potatoes (Chapter 5)
Snack: Pumpkin Pie Apple Slices (Chapter 5)
Dessert: Ginger Mango Sorbet (Chapter 6)

Tuesday (Stage 1)
Breakfast: Blueberry French Toast (Chapter 2)
Lunch: Brown Rice Stir-Fry (Chapter 3)
Dinner: Spaghetti and Meat Sauce (Chapter 4)
Snack: Spicy Baked Tortilla Chips (Chapter 5) with Black Bean Dip (Chapter 5)
Dessert: Pineapple Coconut Popsicles (Chapter 6)

Wednesday (Stage 1)
Breakfast: Mango Pineapple Smoothie (Chapter 2)
Lunch: Savory Bacon and Chive Oatmeal (Chapter 3)
Dinner: Chicken Taco Soup (Chapter 4)
Snack: Quinoa Tabbouleh (Chapter 5)
Dessert: Lemon Mug Cake (Chapter 6)

Thursday (Stage 2)
Breakfast: Bacon and Egg "Muffins" (Chapter 7)
Lunch: Chicken and Egg Salad (Chapter 8)
Dinner: Eggplant Lasagna (Chapter 9)
Snack: Spicy Roast Beef Wraps (Chapter 10)

Friday (Stage 2)
Breakfast: Chicken Sausage with Spinach and Zucchini (Chapter 7)
Lunch: Chicken Burgers (Chapter 8)
Dinner: Pork Roast with Vegetables (Chapter 9)
Snack: Jalapeño Poppers (Chapter 10)

Saturday (Stage 3)
Breakfast: Cacao Power Smoothie (Chapter 11)
Lunch: Cobb Salad (Chapter 12)
Dinner: Coconut Curry Salmon (Chapter 13)
Snack: Guacamole (Chapter 14) with Spicy Baked Tortilla Chips (Chapter 5)
Dessert: Quinoa Pudding (Chapter 15)

Sunday (Stage 3)
Breakfast: Coconut Flour Pancakes with Berry Compote (Chapter 11)
Lunch: Salmon and Spinach Salad with Pumpkin Seeds (Chapter 12)
Dinner: Roasted Chicken with Carrots and Sweet Potatoes (Chapter 13)
Snack: Roasted Chickpeas (Chapter 14)
Dessert: Almond Mug Cake (Chapter 15)

Week 3

Monday (Stage 1)
Breakfast: Chicken Apple Sausage with Scrambled Egg Whites (Chapter 2)
Lunch: Lemon Shrimp with Brown Rice Linguini (Chapter 3)
Dinner: Slow Cooker Adobo Chicken (Chapter 4) with Garlic Zucchini Noodles (Chapter 5)
Snack: Fruit Salad (Chapter 5)
Dessert: Pumpkin Pie Smoothie (Chapter 6)

Tuesday (Stage 1)
Breakfast: Blueberry-Lemon Quinoa Porridge (Chapter 2)
Lunch: Sprouted Tuna Wrap (Chapter 3)
Dinner: Cilantro Lime Chickpea Salad (Chapter 4)
Snack: Pumpkin Pie Apple Slices (Chapter 5)
Dessert: Green Pops (Chapter 6)

Wednesday (Stage 1)

Breakfast: Metabolism-Boosting Smoothie
(Chapter 2)
Lunch: Three-Bean Chili (Chapter 3)
Dinner: Sloppy Joes (Chapter 4) and "Creamed"
Spinach (Chapter 5)
Snack: Baked Grapefruit (Chapter 5)
Dessert: Lemon-Infused Strawberries (Chapter 6)

Thursday (Stage 2)

Breakfast: Spicy Scrambled Eggs (Chapter 7)
Lunch: Cucumber, Tomato, and Tuna Salad
(Chapter 8)
Dinner: Lettuce Wrap Tacos (Chapter 9)
Snack: Dill and Cucumber Salad (Chapter 10)

Friday (Stage 2)

Breakfast: Turkey Bacon and Egg Wrap (Chapter 7)
Lunch: Lemon-Garlic Shrimp with Puréed
Avocado (Chapter 8)
Dinner: Slow Cooker Balsamic Chicken
(Chapter 9)
Snack: Deviled Eggs (Chapter 10)

Saturday (Stage 3)

Breakfast: Sweet Potato Hash with Fried Eggs
and Avocado (Chapter 11)
Lunch: Thai Coconut Spaghetti Squash
(Chapter 12)
Dinner: Quinoa Soup (Chapter 13)
Snack: White Bean Hummus (Chapter 14) with
fresh vegetables
Dessert: Pumpkin Pie Mousse (Chapter 15)

Sunday (Stage 3)

Breakfast: Peach Avocado Smoothie (Chapter 11)
Lunch: Beef and Broccoli Stir-Fry (Chapter 12)

Dinner: Slow Cooker Roast Beef and Mushrooms
(Chapter 13)
Snack: Buffalo Hummus (Chapter 14) with fresh
vegetables
Dessert: Chocolate Coffee Mug Cake (Chapter 15)

Week 4

Monday (Stage 1)

Breakfast: Breakfast Stuffed Sweet Potatoes
(Chapter 2)
Lunch: Mustard-Roasted Salmon (Chapter 3)
Dinner: Garlic Pork Roast (Chapter 4) and
Quinoa Pilaf (Chapter 5)
Snack: Medium apple
Dessert: Blueberry Ginger Smoothie (Chapter 6)

Tuesday (Stage 1)

Breakfast: Amaranth Breakfast Porridge
(Chapter 2)
Lunch: Sweet Potato and Black Bean Burrito
(Chapter 3)
Dinner: Grilled Flank Steak (Chapter 4) and
Balsamic-Glazed Carrots (Chapter 5)
Snack: Fruit Salad (Chapter 5)
Dessert: Blackberry Lemon Sorbet (Chapter 6)

Wednesday (Stage 1)

Breakfast: Vegetable Frittata (Chapter 2)
Lunch: Lemon Chicken Breast (Chapter 3)
Dinner: Pumpkin and Sweet Potato Chili
(Chapter 4)
Snack: Mixed berries
Dessert: Spiced Orange Slices (Chapter 6)

Thursday (Stage 2)
Breakfast: Breakfast Sausage and Peppers (Chapter 7)
Lunch: Shredded Chicken Greek Salad (Chapter 8)
Dinner: Pesto Zucchini "Pasta" (Chapter 9)
Snack: Mediterranean Tomato Salad (Chapter 10)

Friday (Stage 2)
Breakfast: Eggs with Smoked Salmon (Chapter 7)
Lunch: Mini Crab Cakes with Spicy Aioli (Chapter 8)
Dinner: Portobello Burgers (Chapter 9)
Snack: Stuffed Mushrooms (Chapter 10)

Saturday (Stage 3)
Breakfast: Fruit Salad with Coconut Cream (Chapter 11)
Lunch: Hummus and Vegetable Sprouted Wrap (Chapter 12)
Dinner: Curried Chicken Pita (Chapter 13)
Snack: Baked Onion Rings (Chapter 14)
Dessert: Coffee Brownies (Chapter 15)

Sunday (Stage 3)
Breakfast: Stuffed Omelet (Chapter 11)
Lunch: Herbed Broiled Cod (Chapter 12)
Dinner: Spicy Lentil Wraps (Chapter 13)
Snack: Turkey and Avocado Roll-Ups (Chapter 14)
Dessert: Blueberry Granita (Chapter 15)

Week 5

Monday (Stage 1)
Breakfast: Oatmeal Smoothie (Chapter 2)
Lunch: Sardine Salad (Chapter 3)
Dinner: Slow Cooker Lemon Garlic Chicken (Chapter 4) and Summer Squash Bake (Chapter 5)

Snack: Roast Beef and Pickle Wraps (Chapter 5)
Dessert: Baked Cinnamon Apples (Chapter 6)

Tuesday (Stage 1)
Breakfast: Open-Faced Breakfast Sandwich (Chapter 2)
Lunch: Turkey Meatloaf (Chapter 3)
Dinner: Roasted Butternut Squash and Apple Soup (Chapter 4)
Snack: Baked Grapefruit (Chapter 5)
Dessert: Strawberry Kiwi Pops (Chapter 6)

Wednesday (Stage 1)
Breakfast: Cinnamon Pumpkin Smoothie (Chapter 2)
Lunch: Quinoa Summer Squash Salad (Chapter 3)
Dinner: Fish Tacos with Pineapple Salsa (Chapter 4)
Snack: Pumpkin Pie Apple Slices (Chapter 5)
Dessert: Blueberry Lime Sorbet (Chapter 6)

Thursday (Stage 2)
Breakfast: Nutty N'oatmeal (Chapter 7)
Lunch: Roast Beef and Turkey Lettuce Wraps (Chapter 8)
Dinner: Chicken Curry (Chapter 9)
Snack: Avocado Bites (Chapter 10)

Friday (Stage 2)
Breakfast: Frittata with Mixed Greens (Chapter 7)
Lunch: Tuna and Artichoke Salad (Chapter 8)
Dinner: Coconut Shrimp (Chapter 9)
Snack: Buffalo Cauliflower Bites (Chapter 10)

Saturday (Stage 3)
Breakfast: Nutty Oats (Chapter 11)
Lunch: Chicken Vegetable Stir-Fry (Chapter 12)
Dinner: Mediterranean Sweet Potatoes
(Chapter 13)
Snack: Tuna Salad and Cucumber Bites
(Chapter 14)
Dessert: Lemon Bars (Chapter 15)

Sunday (Stage 3)
Breakfast: Chocolate-Covered Blueberry
Smoothie (Chapter 11)
Lunch: Sprouted-Grain BLT (Chapter 12)
Dinner: Quinoa Taco Salad Bowls (Chapter 13)
Snack: Lemon Spinach Artichoke Dip
(Chapter 14) with Spicy Baked Tortilla Chips
(Chapter 5)
Dessert: Vanilla Mug Cake (Chapter 15)

Week 6

Monday (Stage 1)
Breakfast: Turkey Fruit Salad (Chapter 2)
Lunch: Salmon Salad Sandwich (Chapter 3)
Dinner: Pork Chops with Fresh Applesauce
(Chapter 4) and Mashed Parsnips (Chapter 5)
Snack: Baked Grapefruit (Chapter 5)
Dessert: Chocolate Mug Cake (Chapter 6)

Tuesday (Stage 1)
Breakfast: Strawberry Pineapple Smoothie
(Chapter 2)
Lunch: Curried Red Lentil Soup (Chapter 3)
Dinner: Chicken Sausage with Brown Rice Pasta
(Chapter 4)
Snack: Medium apple
Dessert: Spiced Pear Sorbet (Chapter 6)

Wednesday (Stage 1)
Breakfast: Quinoa Breakfast Bowl (Chapter 2)
Lunch: Sun-Dried Tomato, Kale, and Bean Salad
(Chapter 3)
Dinner: Vegetable Rice Soup (Chapter 4)
Snack: Fruit Salad (Chapter 5)
Dessert: Chocolate Coffee Smoothie (Chapter 6)

Thursday (Stage 2)
Breakfast: Sausage Breakfast Muffins (Chapter 7)
Lunch: Salmon with Dill Sauce (Chapter 8)
Dinner: Roasted Chicken (Chapter 9)
Snack: Stuffed Tomatoes (Chapter 10)

Friday (Stage 2)
Breakfast: Avocado Boats (Chapter 7)
Lunch: Stuffed Peppers (Chapter 8)
Dinner: Teriyaki Salmon (Chapter 9)
Snack: Homemade Ranch Dressing (Chapter 10)
with sliced peppers

Saturday (Stage 3)
Breakfast: Root Vegetable Frittata (Chapter 11)
Lunch: Tuna-Stuffed Avocado (Chapter 12)
Dinner: Asian Beef over Wild Rice (Chapter 13)
Snack: Baked Mushrooms (Chapter 14)
Dessert: Cashew Butter Bites (Chapter 15)

Sunday (Stage 3)
Breakfast: Overnight Berry Oatmeal (Chapter 11)
Lunch: Chicken Vegetable Stir-Fry (Chapter 12)
Dinner: Mexican Sweet Potato Casserole
(Chapter 13)
Snack: Sweet Potato Fries (Chapter 14)
Dessert: Chocolate Pudding (Chapter 15)

Resources

The Institute for Functional Medicine
505 S. 336th Street
Suite 600
Federal Way, WA 98003
1-800-228-0622

www.functionalmedicine.org

The goal of the Institute for Functional Medicine is to reverse chronic disease and advance knowledge by providing information and education about functional medicine.

The UltraWellness Center
Dr. Mark Hyman
55 Pittsfield Road
Suite 9
Lenox Commons
Lenox, MA 01240
(413) 637-9991

www.ultrawellnesscenter.com

Dr. Mark Hyman is one of the leaders in functional medicine. He founded the UltraWellness Center in Lenox, Massachusetts, and has authored several books.

Index